Group Therapy
in Independent Practice

Group Therapy in Independent Practice has been co-published simultaneously as *Journal of Psychotherapy in Independent Practice,* Volume 1, Number 2 2000.

Group Therapy
in Independent Practice

Scott Simon Fehr, PsyD
Editor

Group Therapy in Independent Practice has been co-published simultaneously as *Journal of Psychotherapy in Independent Practice,* Volume 1, Number 2 2000.

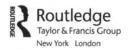

Routledge
Taylor & Francis Group
New York   London

First published by

The Haworth Press, 10 Alice Street, Binghamton, NY 13904-1580

This edition published 2012 by Routledge

Routledge
Taylor & Francis Group
711 Third Avenue
New York, NY 10017

Routledge
Taylor & Francis Group
27 Church Road
Hove East Sussex BN3 2FA

Group Therapy in Independent Practice has been co-published simultaneously as *Journal of Psychotherapy in Independent Practice,* Volume 1, Number 2 2000.

The development, preparation, and publication of this work has been undertaken with great care. However, the publisher, employees, editors, and agents of The Haworth Press and all imprints of The Haworth Press, Inc., including The Haworth Medical Press® and Pharmaceutical Products Press®, are not responsible for any errors contained herein or for consequences that may ensue from use of materials or information contained in this work. Opinions expressed by the author(s) are not necessarily those of The Haworth Press, Inc.

Cover design by Thomas J. Mayshock Jr.

Library of Congress Cataloging-in-Publication Data

Fehr, Scott Simon.
    Group therapy in independent practice / Scott Simon Fehr, editor.
       p. cm.
    Group therapy in independent practice has been co-published simultaneously as Journal of psychotherapy in independent practice, v. 1, no. 2, 2000.
    Includes bibliographical references and index.
    ISBN 0-7890-0758-4 (alk. paper)–ISBN 0-7890-1034-8 (pbk. : alk. paper)
    1. Group counseling. 2. Group psychotherapy. I. Title.
BF637.C6F368 1999
616.89'152–DC21
                                             99-17706
                                               CIP

ABOUT THE EDITOR

Scott Simon Fehr, PsyD, has led over 4000 groups and has had a private practice with his wife, Ellen, for the past 22 years. Dr. Fehr is also Adjunct Faculty with the Masters and APA Approved Doctoral Program in psychology at Nova Southeastern University in Fort Lauderdale, Florida, where he teaches Group and Advanced Group Psychotherapy. Dr. Fehr's other faculty commitments are with the Center for Psychological Studies' Psychodynamic Concentration Program at Nova Southeastern University, and he has taught over the Internet a 12 credit APA continuing education course on group therapy for licensed professionals. He also has supervised license eligible master-level practitioners and post doctoral interns for the past 20 years. Dr. Fehr has been a reviewer for numerous psychology books and journals, and his textbook, *Introduction to Group Therapy: A Practical Guide* has recently been published (The Haworth Press, Inc.). He is a member of the American Group Psychotherapy Association, the American Psychological Association, and the International Association of Group Psychotherapy.

Group Therapy
in Independent Practice

CONTENTS

Introduction to Group Therapy
in Independent Practice

It is with pleasure and excitement that I have been asked to be the editor for this special edition of the *Journal of Psychotherapy in Independent Practice.*

As you are aware, group therapy is a continuing and rapidly growing viable force in the art and practice of psychotherapy. The practice of group therapy in comparison to individual psychotherapy in independent private practices continues to be limited to a small percentage of licensed practitioners although it is a part of almost every in-hospital therapeutic program. Very often it is to be heard that group is a second rate modality in comparison to individual psychotherapy but usually this statement comes from someone who either does not run group or is ignorant to the profound influence group therapy has on personality change. Group is not secondary to any modality and of all the psychotherapeutic interventions utilized by psychotherapists, group therapy most closely resembles real world interactions. Interestingly, the majority of my referrals from other colleagues are for their clients to enter into one of my groups because these practitioners do not implement, for whatever reason(s), group in their own private practices. This creates an opportunity for the private practitioner with group therapy skills another avenue for treating clients' interpersonal difficulties and the possibility of substantial professional economic gains.

In relation to the practice of this modality, group therapy is one of the most naturalistic and therapeutic laboratories for interpersonal learning and relationships. It truly represents a microcosm of the fami-

[Haworth co-indexing entry note]: "Introduction to Group Therapy in Independent Practice." Fehr, Scott Simon. Co-published simultaneously in *Journal of Psychotherapy in Independent Practice* (The Haworth Press, Inc.) Vol. 1, No. 2, 2000, pp. 1-2; and: *Group Therapy in Independent Practice* (ed: Scott Simon Fehr) The Haworth Press, Inc., 2000, pp. 1-2. Single or multiple copies of this article are available for a fee from The Haworth Document Delivery Service [1-800-342-9678, 9:00 a.m. - 5:00 p.m. (EST). E-mail address: getinfo@haworthpressinc.com].

ly, society and civilization. Very few humans live in total isolation by choice but rather interact continuously with members of their society. A vast majority of individuals seeking psychotherapy report that these interactions create feelings of social discomfort, personal alienation, a sense of aloneness and diminished feelings of intimacy with others because of previously unsatisfactory and often repetitively painful emotional experiences. By its very nature, group therapy provides a corrective environment eliciting a two-fold opportunity for these people: an adventure into self-exploration and the possibility of a profound understanding of oneself in relation to humanity and humanity's relationship to oneself.

The following monographs you are about to read have been written by many seasoned clinicians in the arena of group psychotherapy. A diversity of issues is presented in order to hopefully reach the individual personal interests of the reader, e.g., "Personality Disorders: Group Psychotherapy as a Treatment of Choice" by J. Scott Rutan and Cecil A. Rice, "Some Aspects of Intimacy in an Analytic Therapy Group" by Martha Liebmann, "Activity Analysis of Group Process" by Mary Alicia Barnes and Sharan L. Schwartzberg, "Bereavement Groups with the Elderly" by Mark A. Cohen, "Group Psychotherapy and Group Work in Israel–1998" by Haim Weinberg, "The Role of Group Therapy in Promoting Identity Development in ADHD Adolescents" by David Cantor, "Anger in Group Therapy, Countertransference and the Novice Group Therapist" by Steven Van Wagoner, and "An Introduction to the Internet for Independent Group Therapists" by Ralph Cafolla.

I want to thank the many contributors for their time, effort and expertise in their respective fields. It was a pleasure to read your manuscripts; you certainly are a talented group of professionals. I also wish to thank my editorial assistant Sheila Sazant for her invaluable help.

Scott Simon Fehr, PsyD
Hollywood, Florida

Personality Disorders:
Group Psychotherapy
as a Treatment of Choice

J. Scott Rutan, PhD
Cecil A. Rice, PhD

SUMMARY. In past years diagnostic schemata were both simpler and more descriptive. For instance, we distinguished people with "affective" disorders, "thought" disorders, and "personality" disorders. In other words, people had trouble with their feelings, their capacity to think rationally, or with their fundamental personality. The latter is the focus of this paper. *[Article copies available for a fee from The Haworth Document Delivery Service: 1-800-342-9678. E-mail address: getinfo@haworthpressinc.com <Website: http:// www.haworthpressinc.com>]*

KEYWORDS. Personality disorders, group psychotherapy

Dr. Rutan is past president, American Group Psychotherapy Association, Distinguished Fellow, American Group Psychotherapy Association, author, co-author or editor of four books and numerous articles. He is founder of the Center of Group Psychotherapy, Massachusetts General Hospital and Co-Founder of the Boston Institute for Psychotherapy.

Dr. Rice is on the faculties of the Harvard Medical School at Massachusetts General Hospital and Smith College School of Social Work. He is a Fellow of the American Group Psychotherapy Association, Past President of the Northeastern Society for Group, Associate Editor of the International Journal of Group Psychotherapy and Editor of the Bulletin of the Boston Institute for Psychotherapy. Dr. Rice has published numerous articles in the specialty of group psychotherapy and is a Co-founder of Boston Institute of Psychotherapy. Dr. Rice maintains a private practice in Massachusetts.

[Haworth co-indexing entry note]: "Personality Disorders: Group Psychotherapy as a Treatment of Choice." Rutan, J. Scott, and Cecil A. Rice. Co-published simultaneously in *Journal of Psychotherapy in Independent Practice* (The Haworth Press, Inc.) Vol. 1, No. 2, 2000, pp. 3-11; and: *Group Therapy in Independent Practice* (ed: Scott Simon Fehr) The Haworth Press, Inc., 2000, pp. 3-11. Single or multiple copies of this article are available for a fee from The Haworth Document Delivery Service [1-800-342-9678, 9:00 a.m. - 5:00 p.m. (EST). E-mail address: getinfo@haworthpressinc.com].

INTRODUCTION

Classic literary tragedy, according to Grolier's encyclopedia, is *"a drama . . . in which the main character is brought to ruin or suffers extreme sorrow, especially as a consequence of a tragic flaw, a moral weakness, or an inability to cope with unfavorable circumstances."*[1]

For our purposes, we may understand these fallen heroes as individuals suffering from Personality Disorders, though the distinction between some character flaws and psychosis may not be as finely drawn in literature as in the DSM. Literature is rife with examples of such individuals.

For example, when *King Lear* banishes his daughter Cordelia, her fiancé, the King of France, assumes she must have done some monstrous act. So, Cordelia pleads with her father to speak the truth:

I yet beseech your majesty, –
If for I want that glib and oily art,
To speak and purpose not; since what I well intend,
I'll do't before I speak, –that you make known
It is no vicious blot, murder, or foulness,
No unchaste action, or dishonour'd step,
That hath deprived me of your grace and favor; . . .

King Lear:

Better thou
Hadst not been born, than not to have pleased me better.

King of France:

Is it but this? A tardiness in nature,
Which often leaves the history unspoken,
That it intends to do?. . . .
Fairest Cordelia, thou art most rich,
*   being poor;. . . .*
Thee and thy virtues here I seize upon,
. . . I take up what's cast away.

Later Lear's daughters talk among themselves about their father:

Goneril:

. . . he has always loved our sister most; and with what poor judgement he hath cast her off appears too grossly.

Regan:

'Tis the infirmity of his age: yet he hath ever but slenderly known himself.

Goneril:

The best and soundest of his time hath been but rash; then must we look to receive from his age, not alone the imperfections of long engrafted condition, but, therewithal, the unruly waywardness that infirm and choleric years bring with them.[2]

Whose "tardiness of nature" (or Personality Disorder) is really the focus here? Certainly not Cordelia's. It is King Lear whose suspicious and paranoid personality cannot accept that his daughter does not conform to his expectations, his cavernous need for flattery that cannot be filled.

Other examples are Conrad's *Lord Jim*, Dostoevsky's *The Brothers Karamazov*, and Arthur Miller's Willy Loman in *Death of A Salesman*. Truly, a Personality Disorder is a *tragic flaw–a long engrafted condition*.

PERSONALITY DISORDERS

From a psychodynamic perspective, the tragic flaw is a solution to a problem–an ingenious organizing of one's inner life and behavior to manage past and potential overwhelming events, traumas, or perceptions.[3] We wonder what deprivation of love drove King Lear to seek flattery in exaggerated form to fill the emptiness he felt. What given temperament led him to look outside himself rather than within? What lack of comforting inner objects led him to act impulsively rather than bear discomfort? Though we do not know the answer to these questions, we witness the tragic outcome. The "solution" he devised to meet his needs drove away and destroyed what he had and needed most. He lost his daughters and his self-respect. Those who would love him hated him. At the same time, the "solution" *created* the very antipathy he most feared and needed.

People with personality disorders are uniquely difficult to treat because, like King Lear, they often do not perceive a *need* to change. The problems are perceived to be outside themselves. They may not like how life is going, but they do not experience *themselves* as contributing to their difficulties. They often experience their personality as a *given*, predicated on preverbal assumptions that are difficult to assess or evaluate.

> *Once a scorpion and a frog arrived on the bank of a river together. As the frog was about to swim across, the scorpion asked, "Since I cannot swim, would you give me a ride across on your back?"*
>
> *The frog replied, "Of course not!" "You would sting me and I would die." The scorpion countered, "Why should I do that? If I stung you, we would both die, since I would drown."*
>
> *Swayed by the scorpion's logic, the frog agreed to give the spider a ride. Half way across the river the scorpion stung the frog.*
>
> *"Why did you do that?" yelled the frog. "Now we'll both die!"*
>
> *"I know," said the scorpion. "I could not help myself. I'm a scorpion, it's just my nature to sting frogs."*

Besides illustrating the scorpion's uncritical acceptance of the way it is, we can use this story to illustrate another aspect of personality disorders. Arguably, the frog also has a personality disorder; it also uncritically accepts. It is gullible, bringing misery to itself through the action of others. Thus, for our purposes, it can be helpful to place personality disorders on a continuum from active to passive–while acknowledging there are no pure cases. Some people with personality disorders create difficulty in their lives largely because of the pain and misery they inflict on others. These include obsessive-compulsive, borderline and narcissistic disorders. Others create difficulty in their lives by behaving in ways that may cause them to miss opportunities and/or invite others to cause them harm. These include hysterical, passive-dependent, depressive and avoidant personality disorders. Some personality disorders may move back and forth along this continuum, such as passive-aggressive disorders, and some narcissistic and borderline personality disorders can take strongly passive forms.

Not infrequently, people with active or passive style personality disorders find each other. They find each other in work situations, in love relations and in therapy groups. When they find each other, they can create sadomasochistic sexual and/or emotional relationships, dependent and independent struggles and battles over overt and covert power.[4] Like the frog and the scorpion, sometimes they both drown emotionally, and in extreme cases may kill each other. When treating couples, for example, it is almost invariably true that partners complain about their "other" for precisely the reason they *chose* them.

HEALING PROCESSES FOR PERSONALITY DISORDERS IN GROUP THERAPY

Researchers and clinicians alike have long viewed group therapy as a primary treatment for those suffering from Personality Disorders.[5] Group therapy offers many unique advantages for these individuals. The personal style of individuals inevitably shows itself in the interpersonal matrix of the group. Over time the group offers these individuals the opportunity to explore the fantasies and assumptions that fuel their personal style. Additionally, the interpersonal consequences of personal style become highlighted in the group interactions. Foulkes spoke of groups as a "hall of mirrors,"[6] in which the responses that group members receive in a well-functioning group provide invaluable data in assessing the effect of personal style on others.

In addition, Yalom[7] reminds us of the power of *universality* in groups. Most people suffering from a personality disorder feel unique and distinctly alone. In groups they quickly learn that almost *no* human experience or perception cannot be shared by others. This recognition that we are all part of the human community is in and of itself healing. It is especially so for those suffering from personality disorders.

Groups also offer unique opportunities to receive feedback about one's impact on others. This is often referred to as confrontation. Confrontation, however, has a harsh and sometimes pejorative ring to it. We prefer to think of this as a form of mirroring, the opportunity for others to hold up a mirror that accurately reflects aspects of self that may not otherwise be apparent.

Some of the most informative mirroring occurs as members explore their uses of projective identification. As alluded to regarding the tale of the scorpion and the spider, most projective identifications are a multi-person endeavor. There must be a "sender" and a "receiver"; usually the projections go back and forth, amplifying the resonation. Through body language and looks; through the tones, rhythms and cadences of speech; through humor, feelings, mood, behavior, and much else the "sender" (a group member) talks to the "receiver" (other group member/s) and conveys much more than he or she says. These multiple ways of communicating often evoke in the receiver/s a variety of feelings: pleasure, desire, despair, anxiety and anger. They can also evoke unexpected fantasies, thoughts, dreams and nightmares, and effect how they think. These ways of talking are the vehicles of the sender's projections, projecting on to the receiver/s his/her unwanted and frequently unrecognized inner conflicts. These inner conflicts are often referred to as inner object relations because the conflicts usually refer to both remembered and long forgotten conflicts with important people in the sender's life.

Inner object relations are paradoxical in nature. They are montages of relations connected and separated by love and hate, hope and despair, joy and sadness, among many other contradictory phenomena. Thus projective identification describes an unconscious process in which the "sender" "splits-off" unwanted but needed aspects of those paradoxical units. He or she projects them onto one or more "receivers." (Sometimes the projections are also aspects of internal relations the "sender" wishes to protect.) Thus, the experiences evoked in the "receiver" are usually consistent with the "sender's" projections, which the receiver often feels invited to play out.

Not uncommonly the "receivers" of projective identifications project complementary internal relations they wish to disown (the complementary portion of the paradox) on to the original "sender," evoking in them complementary experiences. Usually these projections go back and forth, amplifying and continuously resonating with each other. In time the participating members become locked in an intense repetitive collusion that may on occasion include the therapist. These collusions are usually repetitions of the binds people with Personality Disorders repeat endlessly and seemingly automatically in their daily lives.

The "mirroring" and "confrontation" in the group, especially from the members not caught in a particular collusion, invite those in collusion to examine their contribution to it. Doing this enables them to become aware of aspects of themselves they had previously tried to ignore. Additionally, when a particular collusion is often and adequately reflected on, it can lead the players to accept their unwanted aspects as desirable and valuable.

These collusions that people with Personality Disorders repeat endlessly and seemingly automatically in their daily lives, also reach back to the past. They are the creative acts people with Personality Disorders use to manage the vicissitudes of their early inner and outer environments, however ineffective they may be in the here-and-now. The intensity of group therapy collusions, while seeming like a vivid repetition of that history, also encourage the member to reflect on it, understand its hidden fantasized solution and mourn its loss. The mourning reduces the power of the past, and frees the member to consider other ways of dealing with the same conflicts. Other group members often make available a wide variety of other behaviors to be learned, copied or imitated.[8]

Part of the genius of Projective Identification is that it allows individuals to choreograph their interpersonal world so that others play out expected roles. That is, the individual who has learned to expect that others will be angry and disapproving can "communicate" in ways that evoke angry and critical responses.

CLINICAL EXAMPLE

Bob, a never-married engineer in his 40's, came from an extremely dysfunctional family. His father was a sadistic, alcoholic man who routinely beat his wife and son. These beatings occurred at random times, whether father was drunk or sober. Further, these moments of physical abuse were the only times father seemed to notice Bob at all. This left Bob with a psychological dilemma: either he is neglected and alone in the world or he is the subject of intense abuse. Since any human contact is better than none at all, Bob developed an interpersonal style which invited angry responses. His history included many physical encounters, often with strangers, which he almost always lost.

Charles was the son of a military man. While his father never actually struck Charles, there was an air of imminent physical danger at all times. In order to "toughen up" his son, Charles' father would often punish him by making him do extreme numbers of push-ups or sit-ups. He would jeer at any sign of fear in his son, and he would compliment Charles whenever he was involved in a physical altercation at school.

From the moment they met one another in a therapy group, Bob and Charles had a powerful relationship. They usually sat next to one another despite professing great hatred for one another. Bob would often arrive late, which grated on Charles' need for order and precision. Charles would challenge Bob on his tardiness in bold and aggressive ways, usually looking slyly to the leader for approval.

From a dynamic perspective, Bob was using interpersonal skills developed to gain some connection to father. The cost of this behavior was exorbitant (he could cite almost no examples of being liked by anyone). While he experienced no angry or aggressive feelings of his own, he projected them successfully onto almost everyone in his environment. Charles, on the other hand, was a willing actor in Bob's play. Indeed, he had been trained his whole life to seek his father's attention via aggression. Charles' fears and doubts were unacceptable to him, but he projected them in an interpersonal style which left others frequently feeling fretful, weak and frightened.

This interaction reached a crescendo one evening in group when Bob cavalierly walked in 30 minutes late. Charles glared at him and sat scething but saying nothing. The group fell silent, sensing danger. Bob finally looked at Charles and challenged him, "So what's the matter with *you?*" "You! You're the matter," retorted Charles. Turning to the group leader, Charles inquired, "What are you going to do here? Bob is an unfit group member. He can't follow the rules." Bob incited the situation by saying to Charles, "So, little boy, you want to be daddy's favorite?" "You need a good beating!" replied Charles. "And I'm just the man to give it to you!" With that Charles stood menacingly over Bob and it appeared he would strike him. Bob made no move to defend himself, but sat smiling.

At this point the leader intervened and asked all to notice the body language of the two men–Charles standing with fist clinched and Bob smiling. The leader asked for group associations and immediately one of the members said, "It's like being back home with Bob and Charles. Bob is waiting for father's blows and Charles is trying to prove to his father that he's a good-enough son." Both Bob and Charles were dumbfounded, and first Bob and then Charles began to weep.

CONCLUSION

Certainly not all group interactions with Personality Disorders are as dramatic as that between Bob and Charles. However, groups provide remarkable opportunities to observe the interpersonal world of these patients. In no other setting do we have all the interpersonal data to help these patients connect present behavior to historical antecedents. In no other setting is there such a powerful vehicle for helping these individuals begin to assess *their* contributions to their heartaches.

REFERENCES

1. (1997). *1998* Grolier multimedia encyclopedia. CD version. Danbury, CT: Grolier Interactive, Inc.

2. Shakespeare, W. (1983). King Lear, in The globe illustrated Shakespeare: The complete works annotated. New York: Greenwich House, pp. 1587-1588.

3. Rutan, J.S., Alonso, A., & Groves, J.E. (1998). Understanding defenses in group therapy. *International Journal of Group Psychotherapy, 38* (4): 459-472.

4. Albee, E.F. (1962). Who's afraid of Virginia Woolf.

5. Rutan, J.S., & Stone, W.N. (1993). Psychodynamic group psychotherapy (2nd Ed.). New York: Guilford Publication, Gans, J.S., Alonso A. (1998) Difficult patients: their construction in group therapy. *International Journal of Group Psychotherapy, 48*(3): 311-326.

6. Foulkes, S.H. (1964). Therapeutic group analysis. London: George Allen and Unwin.

7. Yalom, I.D. (1975). The theory and practice of group psychotherapy (2nd Edition). New York: Basic Books, pp. 7-9.

8. Rice, C.A. (1998). Group therapists, poets, and other artists: reflections on God, the devil and projective identification. *The International Journal of Group Psychotherapy, 48*(1): 107-116.

Some Aspects of Intimacy
in an Analytic Therapy Group

Martha Liebmann

SUMMARY. Failure to establish or sustain intimacy is a major reason most patients give for entering therapy, and this is especially so for group therapy. Their hope is that through the here-and-now nature of the group, the peer feedback from the group, and the development of interpersonal dynamics within the group, an atmosphere will be created in which issues of trust and intimacy can be safely explored and worked through. After a brief review of the literature on the subject, case material will be used from the presenter's practice, notably excerpts from a session of a long-term (25 years) analytic therapy group illustrating members' attempts to establish and foster intimacy on the one hand, and to defend against and avoid it, on the other. Discussion will focus on the identification of mechanisms that encourage or deter the development of intimacy. *[Article copies available for a fee from The Haworth Document Delivery Service: 1-800-342-9678. E-mail address: getinfo@ haworthpressinc.com <Website: http://www.haworthpressinc.com>]*

KEYWORDS. Intimacy, interpersonal dynamics, psychoanalytic, psychodynamic, group psychotherapy

---

Dr. Liebmann is a psychoanalytic therapist in private practice in New York and New Jersey. She was trained in ego psychology under the tutelage of the Drs. Blank and in analytic group therapy under the supervision of the Fenchels. Dr. Liebmann has supervised and taught at the Washington Square Institute in New York City and at the Institute for Psychoanalysis and Psychotherapy of New Jersey. She is a certified hypnotherapist and is an Associate Clinical Member of the American Group Psychotherapy Association.

[Haworth co-indexing entry note]: "Some Aspects of Intimacy in an Analytic Therapy Group." Liebmann, Martha. Co-published simultaneously in *Journal of Psychotherapy in Independent Practice* (The Haworth Press, Inc.) Vol. 1, No. 2, 2000, pp. 13-19; and: *Group Therapy in Independent Practice* (ed: Scott Simon Fehr) The Haworth Press, Inc., 2000, pp. 13-19. Single or multiple copies of this article are available for a fee from The Haworth Document Delivery Service [1-800-342-9678, 9:00 a.m. - 5:00 p.m. (EST). E-mail address: getinfo@haworthpressinc.com].

INTRODUCTION

Considering the importance of the concept, there is little written in the literature about the subject of intimacy, and no real attempt to define it. For the purpose of this paper, I would like to use the following definition from an article on object relations by Burgner and Edgcumbe (1972, p. 328): ". . . the capacity to recognize and tolerate loving and hostile feelings toward the same object; the capacity to keep feelings centered on a specific object; and the capacity to value an object for attributes other than its function of satisfying needs."

Analytic group therapy can be both a strengthener of individual identity and the quest for intimacy, as well as a threat to it. The strengthening comes from group support, identification and validation. The threat comes from a weak ego's difficulty in experiencing and reconciling self and other.

The emotional intimacy of any relationship, but especially a group therapy relationship, which confronts individual boundaries in an intense and consistent way, can be especially traumatic to the borderline and/or narcissistic ego. A therapy group member thus challenged will typically strive to maintain his or her boundaries at any cost, even at the risk of alienating the other members. As Ross (1985, p. 724) states in her paper on marital intimacy, "acknowledging the other's needs is seen as involving a denial of the self, that is, giving to others means taking from self, rather than the more mature position that giving to others enhances self." In the same vein, Kernberg (1980, p. 290) asserts that ". . . there can be no meaningful love relation without the persistence of the self, without firm boundaries of the self, which generate a sense of identity."

Kernberg (1980, p. 6) goes on to detail at what interpersonal cost borderline patients, particularly, strive to maintain their ego integrity. In such patients, ". . . splitting, primitive idealization, projective identification, denial, omnipotence and devaluation protect the ego from conflicts by means of dissociating and actively keeping apart contradictory experiences of the self and of significant others. These contradictory ego states are alternately activated, and as long as they can be kept separate from each other, anxiety related to these conflicts is prevented or controlled. However, these defenses, although they protect borderline patients from intrapsychic conflicts, do so at the cost of weakening the patients' ego functioning, thereby reducing their adaptive effectiveness and flexibility."

In an analytic therapy group, where contradictory ego states are constantly being confronted and challenged, it is obvious that major anxieties are going to be summoned and expressed, and done so in the presence of others trying similarly to avoid having their fragile ego integrity abused. Along with the anxiety, comes primitive aggression for (Kernberg, 1980, p. 295) "repressed or dissociated pathogenic object relations from infancy and childhood are reactivated in the context of intimacy throughout time."

Insofar as the conflicts emerging within group process mirror the intrapsychic conflicts of each of the group members, the infighting and avoidance of intimacy must be seen as an expression of incompatible intrapsychic elements that the individual member finds difficult to assimilate. Obviously it requires an atmosphere of great safety for 8 or so group members with varying degrees of borderline pathology, to function, grow, and avoid annihilating one another. Irvin Yalom posits that the core of the borderline's problems lie in the realm of intimacy and that group cohesiveness is the decisive factor in enabling such members to tolerate the group experience. Yalom (1995, p. 402) states that "if the patient is able to accept the reality testing offered by the group, and if his or her behavior is not so disruptive as to create a deviant or scapegoat role, then the group may become a positive holding environment–an enormously important, supportive refuge from the stresses the patient experiences in everyday life." Yalom (1995, p. 231) goes on to say that the curative work of the group may be fostered by the borderline patient's ready access to affect, fantasy, fears and unconscious needs. In his view, problems with intimacy manifest themselves via schizoid withdrawal, fears of aggression against other members, unrealistic demands for instant gratification, fear of self-disclosure and premature self-disclosure.

So far we have concerned ourselves with how borderline patients function in group. What of the narcissistic patient? If borderline patients have fragmented boundaries and need to defend against merging, the narcissistic patients, according to Rutan, Alonso and Groves, (1988, p. 464), ". . . pretend that others are not important. They have a distorted sense of empathy; if they have never felt 'known' they cannot 'know' anyone else. They try desperately not to let either of us understand how important we are to them."

Complicating the whole picture is the fact that defenses in group originate from three different sources, namely, the individual, the group as a whole, and the group therapist's countertransference. This makes for a volatile, unpredictable, and potentially explosive therapeutic situation.

It is also fertile ground for patients' projective identifications, whereby they assign characteristics unacceptable in themselves to other group members, who then act out the despised characteristics. The danger of scapegoating in such an atmosphere is omnipresent, and poses a continual challenge to the group therapist, whose task it is to preserve both the integrity of the group and of each individual within it.

Ironically, their defenses deprive individual group members of the intimacy they crave. As Dugo and Beck point out (1984, p. 30) "as part of the process, they stop others who endeavor to be close to them. The patient with devices to avoid intimacy and to sabotage relationships finds himself forced to deal with those devices–forced both by the nature of the treatment he has agreed to and by the other members."

The above concepts relating to intimacy can be well illustrated by material from a long-term analytic group I have been leading for over 20 years. The group has a unique character derived from the fact that most of its members are creatively inclined. Its membership of 7 at the time this paper was written included 2 musicians, 2 actors, 1 artist, and 2 aspiring writers, ranging in age from 27 to 42. They were all clinic patients, each of whom demonstrated varying degrees of borderline and/or narcissistic pathology. Despite this, the group has had a high degree of cohesion, attendance was good, and there was a feeling of mutual respect and support among the members.

The session I am about to describe happened shortly after the loss of a male member and the introduction of a new male member, Syd, into the group. Syd had been in a prior group which he disliked, but nonetheless was highly enthusiastic about entering this one, hoping it would help him overcome his difficulties in relating to the opposite sex. The following happened during Syd's 5th session in group.

Nina: I've been itching a lot lately. It reminds me of when I was a teenager and I got infested with mites. I went to the doctor and all he told me was to leave them alone and they'd go to someone else.

Syd: I used to have terrible acne, and my doctor gave me painful treatments that didn't help. He had no sympathy.

Liz: I had acne too. I had boils all over my face that were so bad I couldn't leave the house for 2 years. It was like this story I read about a man who went around dressed like a mummy so no one could see his face. I go around wishing no one could look at me.

Shirley: I guess I was lucky. People were always telling me what a pretty child I was. My mother always told them "she knows it." I did know I was pretty, and I still do, but no one wants me.

Liz: You're a great person and I admire you tremendously, Shirley, for your spirit and enthusiasm and passion, but you always come across as so needy, and it turns people off.

Shirley: You really piss me off, Liz. You sit back and look at me like an animal in a zoo, something wild and untamed. You're so condescending, you make me feel like a beast who should be locked up.

Liz: I didn't mean to offend you, but you always pick people who are bound to disappoint you.

Shirley: Well, at least I'm out there trying. You hide in your house and won't let anybody near you. You'll never get love that way.

Liz: I want love too. I just can't risk anyone getting close enough to hurt me.

Therapist: Syd, how do you feel about what is being said?

Syd: I feel like I don't belong here, like I'm on another planet.

Therapist: Which planet is that?

Syd: Mars

Therapist: That's a very warlike planet. Are you very angry?

Syd: No, just disgusted. Nobody listens to me.

Therapist: If they did, what would they hear?

Syd: I think Shirley just doesn't get it.

Shirley: That's the kind of remark my husband always made to me, always putting me down when he was feeling insecure.

Therapist: Are you attracted to Syd, Shirley?

Shirley: Of course. Don't I always get attracted to men who put me down? And Syd does remind me of my husband.

Therapist: Syd, how do you feel about Shirley?

Syd: I find her very attractive. But I can't talk to her. We're on different planets.

Nina: We're all on different planets, but we're in the same galaxy, and we have to establish some kind of intergalactic communication, otherwise we'll all die, because we need to help each other to survive.

Syd: Maybe you're right, but I hate the thought I might need any of you, or that you might need me. I have a powerful urge to leave the group.

Shirley: That's why you belong in this group. We all feel that way. And we're all working on it. You push all my buttons, but I want you to stay here and work with us on making it better.

Syd: I guess I'll come back next week, but no promises after that.

In this session, we see the members' primitive anxieties around merging, abandonment, defectiveness and annihilation, and their desperate attempts to connect and disconnect in an effort to feel whole and lovable. There is already insecurity, anger and helplessness related to the fact that one of the members left, disturbing the integrity of the group. The new member, Syd, is being experienced as an infestation of an alien presence (mites), and a threat to the individual and group boundaries. The doctor (therapist/parent) is seen as indifferent to the problem, and basically leaving everyone to fend for themselves. One solution is to withdraw into a mummy-like (symbiotic) cocoon and pretend the other person isn't there. Another is to attack the invading party and hope they'll either retreat or be conquered. The zoo metaphor represents fears that intimacy will uncage the (id) beasts who will then roam free and inflict great harm upon, perhaps even kill, the object. The "planet Mars" metaphor symbolizes the need to repel attempts at intimacy in order to maintain boundaries and avoid enmeshment. The painful self-disclosures did not lead to the desired instant gratification, as the members struggled to make sense out of their painful experiences and to tentatively reach out to one another despite a certainty that to do so will only lead to more pain and disappointment. As they mirror each others' sense of defectiveness and undesirability, they become aware that choosing a similarly defective partner for intimacy is both inevitable and self-defeating. They want to know they are beautiful and lovable, but all they see are reflections of their own ugliness and hatefulness.

Yet, there is an awareness that they are all they've got, and they'd better learn to deal with each other if they are to survive. Their narcissism would like to deny their importance to each other and their wishes to be nurtured by each other. Their observing egos won't allow them to alienate or abandon each other permanently, because then they would lose any hope of being fed and loved. As Kernberg (1980, p. 127) says, "the tolerance of the limits of one's creativity also tests the sense of inner conviction that love is stronger than hate in one's relations with oneself and with significant others. Normal resolution of this painful learning process increases the capacity to identify with what others create, to experience enjoyment and gratitude rather than jealousy, shame, and envy."

The members of this group, and of countless other groups like it, continue to return week after week in the endless hopeful/fearful search for fulfillment with others. Whether or not they find it is dependent on a willingness to engage in the process of "intergalactic communication" referred to in the session cited. The awareness that the therapist and the other group members can survive the expression of id impulses without significant damage and that the process can engender closeness, trust and a kind of emotional safety, is in itself curative. As Ehrenberg says (1992, p. 67), "sometimes just the discovery that certain kinds of intimacy are possible is significant." Getting past the shame, mistrust, hopelessness and anger to the shared humanity is an essential first step in the quest for intimacy.

REFERENCES

Burgner, M. & Edgcumbe, R., (1972). Some problems in the conceptualization of early object relationships. *Psychoanalytic Study of the Child, 27,* 315-333.

Dugo, J.M., and Beck, A.P., (1984). A therapist's guide to issues of intimacy and hostility viewed as group-level phenomena. *International Journal of Group Psychotherapy, 38,*1, 29-46

Ehrenberg, D.B., (1992). The intimate edge. New York: W.W. Norton, Inc.

Kernberg, O., (1980). Internal world and external reality. New York: Jason Aronson.

Ross, J.L., (1985). Intimacy, boundaries and identity in marriage. *Psychotherapy, 22,*4, 724-728.

Rutan, J.S., Alonso, A., and Groves, J.F., (1988). Understanding defenses in group psychotherapy. *International Journal of Group Psychotherapy, 38,* 4, 459-472

Yalom, I.D., (1995). The theory and practice of group psychotherapy. New York: Basic Books.

Activity Analysis of Group Process

Mary Alicia Barnes
Sharan L. Schwartzberg

SUMMARY. There are a variety of theoretical models accepted within the practice of group psychotherapy. These approaches include interpersonal, intrapsychic, and behavioral methods. The focus on here-and-now versus there-and-then varies. It is often determined by the leader's clinical training and demands of the setting relative to reimbursement factors. Regardless of these factors a match must be made between the member's ability to func-

---

Mary Alicia Barnes, OTR/L, has been practicing in the field of occupational therapy with adolescents with chronic and persistent mental illness and forensic psychiatric issues for 12 years. She assists in teaching and coordinating fieldwork education at Tufts University-Boston School of Occupational Therapy. She has published on subject areas of clinical education, occupational therapy in child and adolescent psychiatry, and vocational group programming for adolescents with severe emotional disturbance.

Dr. Schwartzberg is Professor and Chair of the Boston School of Occupational Therapy at Tufts University, Graduate School of Arts and Sciences. She is Associated Staff in the departments of Psychiatry and Occupational Therapy at Mount Auburn Hospital, Cambridge, Massachusetts. She teaches courses in Group Therapy and supervises student research. Dr. Schwartzberg has published several chapters, articles and books in occupational therapy. Her book, co-authored with Margot Howe, is now being revised for a third edition. She is particularly recognized for scholarship in the area of peer support for individuals of post traumatic head injury. Currently her research includes a study of the interactive reasoning process in occupational therapy to be a published in her forthcoming book.

The first author would like to thank her colleagues and coleaders, Jim Judkins and Lisa Lindberg, at the UMASS Adolescent Inpatient Program, Westboro, MA, as well as, her colleague and mentor Sharan L. Schwartzberg, without whom this work would not be possible.

[Haworth co-indexing entry note]: "Activity Analysis of Group Process." Barnes, Mary Alicia, and Sharan L. Schwartzberg. Co-published simultaneously in *Journal of Psychotherapy in Independent Practice* (The Haworth Press, Inc.) Vol. 1, No. 2, 2000, pp. 21-32; and: *Group Therapy in Independent Practice* (ed: Scott Simon Fehr) The Haworth Press, Inc., 2000, pp. 21-32. Single or multiple copies of this article are available for a fee from The Haworth Document Delivery Service [1-800-342-9678, 9:00 a.m. - 5:00 p.m. (EST). E-mail address: getinfo@haworthpressinc.com].

tion and the group process activity. *[Article copies available for a fee from The Haworth Document Delivery Service: 1-800-342-9678. E-mail address: getinfo@haworthpressinc.com <Website: http://www.haworthpressinc.com>]*

KEYWORDS. Group process, group psychotherapy, activity analysis

INTRODUCTION

Recent studies demonstrate adverse outcomes when the relationship between level of psychopathology and social structure such as group work roles are misaligned (Greene & Cole, 1991). Patients' perceptions of therapeutic dimensions of group psychotherapy and occupational therapy (Eklund, 1997; Falk-Kessler, Momich, & Perel, 1991; Finn, 1989; Schwartzberg, Howe, & McDermott, 1982; McDermott, 1988; Webster & Schwartzberg, 1992) have been differentiated by activity analysis. The myth of verbal activity being related to therapeutic outcomes has also been called into question (Soldz, Budman, Demby, & Feldstein, 1990).

ACTIVITY ANALYSIS OF GROUP PROCESS

Activity analysis can help a leader facilitate a positive match between group psychotherapy tasks and capabilities of the individual and the group as a whole (Howe & Schwartzberg, 1995). The process requires a study of the group format prior to initiating a group and as the group progresses.

ACTIVITY ANALYSIS

In occupational therapy three domains (see Figure 1) are mainly addressed in activity analysis: occupational performance areas, performance components, and performance contexts (American Occupational Therapy Association, 1996). Activity adaptation is the process by which a therapist alters the task or environment to enable successful performance. In an activity analysis the therapist seeks to understand the demands placed on an individual in order to function in various activities or contexts. The areas of performance include activities of daily living, work and productive activities, and play or leisure. In order to know the complexity of a task the therapist must identify human and nonhuman demands in performance component areas that include sensorimotor, cognitive, psychosocial, and psychological skills.

ACTIVITY ADAPTATION

All activity is embedded in a context. In the analysis the context influencing desired or required performance needs to be identified. This includes both temporal and environmental aspects. For example, a group member with mobility problems may require space for a wheelchair in the circle of seats. Cultural orientation may require definition of symbols used in communication such as greetings.

A person's place in the lifecycle, such as important life phases in parenting or schooling, help to prioritize therapeutic goals. Disability status, such as adjusting to chronic mental illness, suggests an intervention aimed at altering the context to improve performance rather than characterological change.

REASONING PROCESS

Leader Role

The leader can adjust interventions on the basis of needs of the members. This is more typically thought about and addressed in psychological domains than in cognitive. Needless to say patients come with a variety of attention spans, abilities in the realm of the abstract, and so forth. Therefore, the length of a meeting, number of sessions, depth of content, degree of insight, and ability to learn, remember or problem solve, are some areas to consider when addressing member needs.

Member Selection and Group Composition

The degree of member homogeneity varies depending upon the group model, setting and methods of reimbursement. It is a good idea to analyze the nature of the group process to see that there is a "good-

FIGURE 1. Uniform Terminology for Occupational Therapy, Third Edition Outline (AOTA, 1996)

I. Performance Areas
A. Activities of Daily Living
 1. Grooming
 2. Oral Hygiene
 3. Bathing/Showering
 4. Toilet Hygiene
 5. Personal Device Care
 6. Dressing
 7. Feeding and Eating
 8. Medication Routine Cultural
 9. Health Maintenance
 10. Socialization
 11. Functional Communication
 12. Functional Mobility
 13. Community Mobility
 14. Emergency Response
 15. Sexual Expression
B. Work and Productive Activities
 1. Home Management
  a. Clothing Care
  b. Cleaning
  c. Meal Preparation/
  d. Shopping
  e. Money Management
  f. Household Maintenance
  g. Safety Procedures
 2. Care of Others
 3. Educational Activities
 4. Vocational Activities
  a. Vocational Exploration
  b. Job Acquisition
  c. Work or Job Performance
  d. Retirement Planning
  e. Volunteer Participation
C. Play or Leisure Exploration
 1. Play/Leisure Exploration
 2. Play/Leisure Performance

II. Performance Components
A. Sensorimotor Component
 1. Sensory
  a. Sensory Awareness
  b. Sensory Processing
   (1) Tactile
   (2) Proprioceptive
   (3) Vestibular
   (4) Visual
   (5) Auditory 3.
   (6) Gustatory
   (7) Olfactory
  c. Perceptual Processing
   (1) Stereognosis
   (2) Kinesthesia
   (3) Pain Response
   (4) Body Scheme
   (5) Right-Left Discrimination
   (6) Form Constancy
   (7) Position in Space
   (8) Visual-Closure Cleanup
   (9) Figure Ground
   (10) Depth Perception
   (11) Spatial Relations
   (12) Topographical Orientation
 2. Neuromusculoskeletal
  a. Reflex
  b. Range of Motion
  c. Muscle Tone
  d. Strength
  e. Endurance
  f. Postural Control
  g. Postural Alignment
  h. Soft Tissue Integrity
 3. Motor
  a. Gross Coordination
  b. Crossing the Midline
  c. Laterality
  d. Bilateral Integration
  e. Motor Control

III. Performance Contexts
A. Temporal Aspects
 1. Chronological
 2. Developmental
 3. Life Cycle
 4. Disability Status
B. Environmental Aspects
 1. Physical
 2. Social

f. Praxis
g. Fine Coordination/Dexterity
h. Visual-Motor Integration
i. Oral-Motor Control
B. Cognitive Integration and Cognitive Components
1. Level of Arousal
2. Orientation
3. Recognition
4. Attention Span
5. Initiation of Activity
6. Termination of Activity
7. Memory
8. Sequencing
9. Categorization
10. Concept Formation
11. Spatial Operations
12. Problem Solving
13. Learning
14. Generalization
C. Psychosocial Skills and Psychological Components
1. Psychological
   a. Values
   b. Interests
   c. Self-Concept
2. Social
   a. Role Performance
   b. Social Conduct
   c. Interpersonal Skills
   d. Self-Expression
3. Self-Management
   a. Coping Skills
   b. Time Management
   c. Self-Control

Taken from: American Occupational Therapy Association. (1996). Reference manual of the official documents of the American Occupational Therapy Association, p. 278, 6th Ed. Bethesda, MD: AOTA. Copyright 1996 by the American Occupational Therapy Association, Inc. Reprinted with permission. (Adopted by the AOTA Representative Assembly July 1994.)

ness of fit" between members and the expectations of the group. The analysis should take into consideration performance components that may affect members' ability to function in a group therapy context and what role leaders may need to take to accommodate member needs versus group needs.

Activity Selection, Format and Process

There are various degrees of freedom in activity selection, format and process in various clinical settings. Analysis of the format enables the leader to modify both the human, therapeutic relationships and the nonverbal activity components. In occupational therapy, the "person-activity-environment fit refers to the match among the skills and abilities of the individual; the demands of the activity; and the characteristics of the physical, social, and cultural environments. It is the interaction among the performance areas, performance components, and the performance contexts that is important and determines the success of the performance" (American Occupational Therapy Association, 1996, pp. 276-277). In a verbal group psychotherapy format there are several nonverbal processes that bear activity analysis and examination. The following examples serve to demonstrate the reasoning involved when activity analysis is applied.

Clinical Applications

The following two case examples are from a weekly self awareness group held on an adolescent, long-term inpatient hospital milieu. The group composition is designed to be inclusive of all members of the milieu who have not yet achieved community based privilege. Therefore, the group size and membership fluctuates based on patient status. Group size can vary from 4-14 members. This membership criteria results in a variation of age (12-19 years), level of functioning, level of acuity/safety (safety status to unlocked areas) and attendance and duration of time as a member of the group (1 week to 12 months or more).

Members present with multiple performance problems that span activities of daily living, work, and play/leisure areas. The problems often stem from deficits in performance components (sensory, neuromuscular, motor, cognitive and psychosocial). Members may appear to be functioning developmentally in a manner more typical of a chronologically younger child. The children are at a variety of points on a continuum of understanding their disability status (first hospitalization versus history of mental health services).

The group session is 45 minutes and currently involves a three way coleadership to ensure adequate client to staff ratios, supervision and safety/limit setting. Although membership is considered voluntary, the milieu's behavioral structure allows patients to earn points toward privileges for attendance. Patients who choose not to attend are asked to go to their room. Exclusion criteria include the patient being deemed unsafe by the RN/nursing staff or on a safety precaution that would prohibit being in the milieu at the time of group. In such a situation the child is in a quiet room, restraint, or being evaluated via room time as to readiness to return to milieu program.

Leaders combine behavioral, developmental, psychodynamic and cognitive behavioral approaches in their structure, format and leadership. Due to the variation in ages and functional abilities, a combination of task and verbal media are chosen. The variety allows for differing levels of understanding of the issues and topic, as well as, provides multiple options for self-expression. The emphasis of the group is on increasing understanding of oneself and others to promote greater interdependence and ability to function and relate in a safe, healthy fashion in a community setting.

Each week the group has an opening ritual that reviews the purpose of the group and the rules regarding expectations around participation and behaving in an age appropriate manner. This serves as a group contract that was once devised by the group and must be honored. It outlines the need to listen to others, be open to differences and to engage with others in a safe, mature and respectful fashion. Group norms focus on support, teamwork, tolerance of diversity, nonviolent forms of self-expression and communication.

Yalom's (1983) principles, such as instillation of hope, universality, corrective recapitulation of the primary family group, imitative behavior, cohesiveness, and interpersonal learning, are all therapeutic values integral to the clinical reasoning, leadership and success of the group process.

CASE #1:
BOY WITH COGNITIVE IMPAIRMENT

Andy is a 17 year old white male who has been in multiple residential and foster care placements since age three years. He has a history of physical and sexual abuse. He has been physically aggressive and has attempted suicide on multiple occasions. He reports gang involvement, substance abuse, and is on probation for assault.

Andy's IQ is in the borderline range (V: 85 P: 87: FS 85). He has language based learning disabilities which involve difficulty with auditory processing, and problems with long- and short-term memory. These cognitive deficits affect Andy's ability to perform in school and work contexts, especially with tasks that require reading and writing. Andy also has a visual impairment and gross motor problems that affect his task performance and social skills. For example, he has an awkward gait, will often bump into walls, and stands at a close physical proximity to others. He requires extra time and assistance in the form of verbal cues to attend to details and complete tasks.

Psychological testing indicates that he has low self-worth and violent fantasies. Andy was noted to be vulnerable to manipulation by others, as well as, to risk disappointment in others leading to feelings of rage. Andy's aggression is most directed at those he feels are interfering with his wanting to do what he wants when he wants.

In group, Andy is noted to be loud and is hyperactive but engageable and redirectable. He has difficulty when the group is less structured and requires one to one assistance from the coleader to facilitate his understanding the group's immediate task and goals. He responds well to structured psychoeducational and cognitive behavioral approaches and to semi-structured, expressive art media.

Andy is aware of his issues of behavioral dyscontrol. In this group setting and structure he can be reflective and identify his needs and strengths. To facilitate his remaining in group he needs encouragement, as well as repeated reminders and reinforcement as to what the expectations are around his behavior and participation.

Andy responds well in the group structure to a limit setting approach that focuses on his valuable role as a group member and maintains the group contract by referring to the rules regarding expectations and group member's participating maturely and respectfully. Leaders provide Andy cues and feedback to help him self-monitor his noise/activity level and the content of conversation/verbalizations. In addition, leaders provide suggestions and strategies to manage peer interactions and frustration. Leaders will often give verbal reframes to Andy's self denigrating remarks.

These interactions help him identify affect and decrease distorted thinking. The interventions facilitate Andy's adaptation by allowing him to learn and use more rational problem-solving approaches to managing his affect in task or social situations that emerge in the group.

Within the context of the group process and activities Andy has been able to use structured, expressive art tasks. These have included activities such as drawing in which he characterized his current life situation as "a battlefield" and his wish that he could be "on top of the world."

After several weeks of participation in group Andy was able to take a leadership role in the group during a collective poetry writing session. Initially leaders adopted member roles and role modeled brainstorming ideas for content in a poem about the season. During this process Andy identified himself as a poet. He began writing and reading out loud to the group short simple poems on the topics of spring, his loneliness, and his love of rock and roll music.

Leader's Clinical Reasoning

Andy demonstrates impairments in the sensorimotor, cognitive, and psychological performance components. In this example, the leaders modify their approach and expectations to facilitate Andy's successful functioning as a group member. Through external cues and limits, they adapt their therapeutic use of self to provide absent overseeing or executive cognitive functions such as the ability to initiate, problem solve, and self-monitor. Frequent use of reminders and other carefully timed interventions provide a social map via role modeling and verbal cues. Through these modifications, Andy's psychosocial skills (social conduct and interpersonal interactions) are enhanced. He can perform in a manner to fulfill group norms. Both verbal and nonverbal media are also provided to facilitate expression. In doing so, Andy's remaining strengths and capacities for insight, self-reflection, and self-expression are tapped. He is provided with a meaningful temporal (chronologically age appropriate) and environmental (social and adolescent culture) context for growth and potential change.

CASE #2:
GIRL WITH PTSD, WITH SOME QUESTION
OF BORDERLINE OR NARCISSISTIC
PERSONALITY FEATURES

Kate is an 18 year old female with a history of multiple out-of-home placements and hospitalizations since age 12. She has a history of physical and sexual abuse, self harm and suicide attempts. She presents with learning disabilities and memory problems secondary to a seizure disorder which appears to be the sequellae of a serious drug overdose that resulted in her being in a coma.

Psychological testing indicates longstanding anaclytic depression, and symptomatology suggestive of PTSD, with some question of Borderline or Narcissistic Personality features. Kate is noted to be sadistic in her use of suicidal threats and gestures toward family and caretakers. For example, having made significant suicide attempts in response to limits set by mother, she secretly engaged in self-harm during therapy sessions by tying shoelaces tightly around her neck. She hid this fact by wearing a turtleneck shirt.

In group Kate vacillates between being nonverbal and withdrawn to engaging and demonstrating role model or leadership behavior. At times she will suggest ideas for the group and review out loud the group contract as part of the group's opening ritual. During expressive art tasks Kate often would become very involved with her work and artistically develop images or scenes that would serve as metaphors for her affective state. When tasks were more of a verbal or written nature, Kate would become increasingly anxious and often state she didn't understand or was confused.

On other occasions, she would present as shutdown, bringing a teddy bear to group which she would hug while rocking. During these more regressed states Kate would often refuse to engage in the group task or process, becoming alternatively needy of leader attention, or easily enraged by leader or other member attempts to engage or redirect her. During these times coleader consistency and support with feedback and limit setting was crucial. Kate would need gentle reminders regarding the group contract and her value to the group as a member. However, at times she would be asked to leave the group for that week due to her regressed or disruptive behavior and asked to try to rejoin the following week.

Minimal processing of Kate's behavior or outbursts would occur during or outside of group. To do so appeared to feed into a cycle of negative attention seeking for the leaders' undivided attention. The leaders acknowledged other members for their efforts and caring when they attempted to engage Kate while she was having difficulty in the group. However, the members were then asked to give Kate time and space to learn to struggle safely with her issues. The leaders would express aloud their hope that the group as a whole could find ways to be supportive and communicate with Kate. But they would also maintain the group contract by reiterating the expectations around being able to function, therefore, to participate maturely and respectfully. Furthermore, the leaders reinforced concepts of group safety and holding environment. They reminded members that they did not deserve to nor would leaders tolerate their being subject to Kate's actions and attitude that were verbally or emotionally abusive.

Leader's Clinical Reasoning

Understanding Kate's illness experience in terms of the performance areas, components, and contexts guides the leaders' interventions and reinforcement of the group as a holding environment. Kate appears to use the group as a context in which to struggle with her issues about her disability status and the expectations of the group (age appropriate behavior, use of peer elements in the group's socio-cultural context). This challenges her ability to maintain self-control in light of her extreme neediness and experience of emptiness. Her cognitive and psychosocial skill deficits add to her distress. They directly impair her ability to socialize and communicate when she is overwhelmed or flooded by affect. Her illness makes her alliances fragile. For these reasons, for Kate, the consistency and structure of both the leaders and the group process, contract/norms, and member response are so critical.

CONCLUSIONS

The importance of matching the person, activity, and environment has been illustrated through case examples. Through activity analysis and adaptation group leaders can modify the group process to better achieve therapeutic aims.

REFERENCES

American Occupational Therapy Association. (1996). Reference manual of the official documents of the American Occupational Therapy Association, 6th ed. Bethesda, MD: AOTA.

Eklund, M. (1997). Therapeutic factors in occupational group therapy identified by patients discharged from a psychiatric day centre and their significant others. Occupational Therapy International, 4(3), 198-212.

Falk-Kessler, J., Momich, C., & Perel, S. (1991). Therapeutic factors in occupational therapy groups. *American Journal of Occupational Therapy, 45*(1), 59-66.

Finn, M. (1989). Patients' perceptions of occupational therapy groups: Interview generated factors. Unpublished master's thesis, Tufts University-Boston School of Occupational Therapy.

Greene, L. R., & Cole, M. B. (1991). Level and form of psychopathology and the structure of group therapy. *International Journal of Group Psychotherapy, 41*(4), 499-521.

Howe, M. C., & Schwartzberg, S. L. (1995). A functional approach to group work in occupational therapy, 2nd ed. Philadelphia: J. B. Lippincott.

McDermott, A. A. (1988). The effect of three group formats on group interaction patterns. Occupational therapy in Mental Health: *A Journal of Psychosocial Practice and Research, 8*(3), 69-89.

Schwartzberg, S. L., Howe, M. C., & McDermott, A. (1982). A comparison of three treatment group formats for facilitating social interaction. Occupational therapy in Mental Health: *A Journal of Psychosocial Practice and Research, 2*(4), 1-16.

Soldz, S., Budman, S., Demby, A., & Feldstein, M. (1990). Patient activity and outcome in group psychotherapy: New Findings. *International Journal of Group Psychotherapy, 40*(1), 53-62.

Yalom, I. D. (1983). Inpatient group psychotherapy New York: Basic Books.

Webster, D., & Schwartzberg, S. L. (1992). Patients' perceptions of curative factors in occupational therapy groups. Occupational therapy in mental health: *A Journal of Psychosocial Practice and Research, 12*(1), 3-24.

Bereavement Groups with the Elderly

Mark A. Cohen

SUMMARY. Grief and bereavement are issues that affect almost all of us at some time. The elderly are a group in particular that is strongly affected by bereavement. One out of every elderly couple will eventually lose his/her spouse. Based upon my work with the elderly in bereavement groups, a pattern of what the group provides that is therapeutic to the individual has emerged. These curative factors are the instillation of hope, acceptance, a decrease in social isolation, finding of a new identity and meaning in life, support, catharsis, amelioration of fears, education, assistance in processing and dealing with painful or intense feelings, and an opportunity to help others. These factors and their manifestation in the elderly bereavement group are discussed. *[Article copies available for a fee from The Haworth Document Delivery Service: 1-800-342-9678. E-mail address: getinfo@haworthpressinc.com <Website: http://www.haworthpressinc.com>]*

KEYWORDS. Geriatric, elderly, group psychotherapy, bereavement, mourning

INTRODUCTION

Grief and bereavement are issues that affect most individuals, especially the elderly population. One member of every elderly couple will have to deal with the loss of his/her spouse.

Dr. Cohen completed his post doctoral residency at the Akron Child Guidance Center. His area of specialty is group therapy in relation to many diverse populations. He is supervisor of psychological testing at NorthEast Ohio Health Services, a community mental health center, and consults to three hospitals for psychological services in Ohio. He maintains a private practice which includes individual, group, forensic, and disability evaluations. He also has begun a very successful program of bringing psychotherapy into the homes of elderly patients who could not be seen in an office due to ambulatory disabilities.

[Haworth co-indexing entry note]: "Bereavement Groups with the Elderly." Cohen, Mark A. Co-published simultaneously in *Journal of Psychotherapy in Independent Practice* (The Haworth Press, Inc.) Vol. 1, No. 2, 2000, pp. 33-41; and: *Group Therapy in Independent Practice* (ed: Scott Simon Fehr) The Haworth Press, Inc., 2000, pp. 33-41. Single or multiple copies of this article are available for a fee from The Haworth Document Delivery Service [1-800-342-9678, 9:00 a.m. - 5:00 p.m. (EST). E-mail address: getinfo@haworthpressinc.com].

Not only do elderly individuals eventually lose their spouse or life partner, but there is also the loss of close friends, contemporaries, business partners, neighbors and relatives. However, despite the fact that so many elderly individuals are affected by bereavement, there have not been many articles published focusing on bereavement groups with elderly individuals. The purpose of this article is to discuss the benefits of bereavement groups for the elderly and why it is an effective modality of treatment.

The elderly individual who loses a spouse is confronted with many difficult issues. There are feelings of sadness, guilt, anger, despair, and helplessness. There is sometimes the question of "why?" There is the feeling of "How can I go on?" So what can a bereavement group offer elderly individuals? Yalom (1975), in his textbook on group therapy, talks about the "curative factors" of therapy. Through my work with the elderly in bereavement groups a pattern of what the group provides that is therapeutic to the individual has emerged. These factors are the instillation of hope, acceptance, a decrease in social isolation, finding of a new identity and meaning in life, support, catharsis, amelioration of fears, education, assistance in processing and dealing with painful or intense feelings, and an opportunity to help others.

One of the most obvious things that a bereavement group can bring to elderly individuals is social support. Widowed individuals tend to have good social supports from family and friends during the initial three to four weeks of bereavement, but after that the support tends to wane (Silverman, MacKenzie, Pellipas, & Wilson, 1974). Some group members speak of the fact that when the effect of their loss on other people in their lives dies down and friends stop coming around and calling as much there is a great sense of loneliness. Other individuals report that friends and acquaintances seem to purposefully come around less, almost out of a fear that if they spend time with the bereaved such a tragedy could also befall them. Or, at least it reminds them of their own vulnerability to such a loss and frightens them so they avoid having to confront their own fears. One recently widowed elderly woman reported that her elderly brother-in-law was actually afraid to be around her for fear that she somehow carried death and would cause him to die. Some elderly individuals have limited families and their spouse was their only form of support. The social support that a bereavement group can provide helps to decrease the feelings of loneliness and isolation that elderly individuals often experience.

In addition to social support, a bereavement group can provide acceptance. Individuals report that after time they begin to feel their bereavement is not being accepted by their family and friends. Some bereaved individuals speak of their family and friends telling them to stop crying and to "get over it already!" Society sends the message that they need to stop crying and should not grieve, or at least, should grieve by themselves, perhaps because being around one who is grieving causes us to have to look at our own mortality and vulnerability. The group provides a safe haven where the bereaved can be themselves amongst people who can understand them. As we know, when a bereaved individual stuffs his/her feelings inside this can lead to later complications in the bereavement process. So, providing the bereaved individual with a place where she can express her grief and sorrow without judgment can be freeing and therapeutic for the individual. Being able to release her tears that may have been pent up can be a cathartic experience.

Being amongst people who have shared the same experience and can understand cannot be over emphasized. Group members have stated that their family members have gotten very upset at them when they have said that they feel like they don't want to live anymore. Their family members fear this means the person is going to kill himself. Bereaved individuals have found it a relief to be able to tell others in group that "I just don't feel like living without my spouse" as a way to express their grief without having to worry about a family member telling them "Stop saying that." When they are responded to with support and acceptance of their feelings, it furthers the bereavement process.

When the group setting becomes a safe haven for self-expression without fear of judgment the healing process can begin. I often bring, or have other group members bring into the group, poems that they have found about bereavement, life, love, and healing. Reading of the poems leads to many tears in the group and a feeling of catharsis. It may trigger emotions that the individual is otherwise unable to access. Then there is discussion about how the members can relate to the poems. What is interesting is that many members find and bring in poems that have an uplifting theme. They will speak of terrible sadness and loss but then about the strength of the individual to go on and live another day. Members gain much strength from these poems as they affect them deeply emotionally. Some members have even taken to writing their own poems as a way to express their feelings.

One of the most powerful curative factors of the bereavement group appears to be the instillation of hope; the hope that things can get better, the hope that, with time, the pain and aching in the heart will lessen, the hope that they will one day be able to smile and to enjoy life again. A benefit of the group setting is that newer members or members who are less far along in the bereavement process can observe members who are farther along in the process. They can observe that things can get better. Roy and Sumpter (1983) observed this in their bereavement groups and felt it was an important curative factor. Another benefit of the group setting is that the group can give individuals positive encouragement and support for making difficult changes or trying difficult things. Sometimes members are unable to see the progress they have been making until it is pointed out by group members. For example, one woman cried through every session for many months and then did not even realize she had stopped crying continually until another member pointed it out to her. Having others in group also allows members to see how far they have come because eventually someone will enter the group who is in a stage of bereavement that they have already worked through.

According to Sanders (1989), groups can offer bereaved individuals three types of support: Instrumental support, Emotional support, and Validational support. The first, instrumental support, consists of the giving of ideas on how to handle practical matters based upon one's own experiences. Grief stricken individuals will often feel confused or overwhelmed about how to handle everything from funeral or stone setting arrangements to how to change a light bulb or balance a check book. Individuals in the group who have already handled these matters can discuss what it was like for them, what the options are, and help the individual to make a choice. The newly bereaved find that there are things in their life that their spouse always handled and they may not know how to do them. In one of my bereavement groups a powerful moment came when a woman who thought she could not do many household tasks realized that she had actually learned how to do them just because she had watched her husband do them for many years. Besides giving her a renewed sense of competence in her ability to take care of herself, it also eased her sense of loss by providing her with a feeling that she had internalized parts of her husband's personality.

Other types of instrumental support can range from discussing ways that each has found to deal with the loneliness, such as leaving a radio or television on so that sound fills the room, to discussing what to do with their spouses' clothes and possessions. One common discussion in the bereavement groups is how to deal with other couples and not feel like a "fifth wheel." Members decided that it was important to not let other couples pay for them and that they needed to pay for themselves in order not to feel dependent. They all had to deal with the reality that it is difficult for a single individual to fit into their old world that was mostly couples. They also discussed how married women would start to see them as a threat to their marriage. The advice that members were able to give others about their experiences in these situations and the ability for members to discuss these things and find out they were not alone in their experiences, that it was not just them who seemed to be getting less invitations out by couple friends, was helpful to members.

The second type of support is emotional support and this is the majority of the grief work. The group provides emotional support by listening to the bereaved individual and allowing him/her to repeatedly discuss the death without being judgmental. The group allows the individual to cry and express his/her feelings freely which facilitates the grief process. The group members can provide empathy in that they can relate to the experiences and have been through the same things. The group also provides emotional support by helping the individual to discuss and process difficult emotions.

One powerful emotion that often arises in many forms in the elderly bereavement group is guilt. This emotion ranges from guilt over being alive, guilt over how they handled issues over resuscitation, and guilt over funeral arrangements to guilt over how much they expressed their love to their spouse in life. After years of proving loving support, help, and care taking to their ill spouse, an individual may focus on one thing, such as if they should have had the doctors turn off the respirator a day earlier or which casket they picked, and be racked with guilt about this. This need to blame themselves for something may give them a sense of control over a situation which they had little control over (death). Their guilt may also be a defense against their anger that despite the fact that they did so much for their loved one, he/she still died. The group is a powerful medium to handle issues of guilt. I have found that what the other members say carries much more weight than what the therapist says because the other members have been through it themselves. They can relate to having those same feelings of guilt in the same situations and can help members to test the reality of those thoughts.

Another strong emotion that arises in the groups is anger. The anger may range from very concrete, such as being angry at a spouse who was an alcoholic and died of cirrhosis of the liver or who was a smoker and died of lung cancer despite urgings from doctors to quit, to the more existential, being angry at life, fate, or god. The anger may be directed at the loved one, doctors, family, friends or oneself. In a group setting the anger may be transferred onto another group member who reminds the individual of his/her spouse. For example, an elderly woman whose husband died because he refused to get medical treatment for his heart condition gets extremely angry with a group member who is neglecting their physical health.

The third type of support is validational support. This consists of the group normalizing the grieving process to members and letting them know what to expect. This type of support helps to decrease group members' fears. Often the bereaved fear they are "going crazy" because they will think they see or hear their spouse, cannot remember things said to them, become confused, and have difficulty concentrating. The group can assure the individual that all of these are normal reactions to the grieving process and with time will dissipate. One woman in a group who learned to drive after her husband died used to look up and speak to him after she parked the car and ask him "Did I park the car okay?" She was not expecting an answer but was afraid that her talking to her deceased husband meant she was crazy. Another woman feared she was crazy because in the mornings she liked to put on her husband's bathrobe and could almost feel him hugging her while the robe was wrapped around her.

In bereavement groups there is an opportunity to provide grieving people with education about relevant issues. Both the therapist and other group members can educate members about the stages of bereavement, common symptoms, and what to expect as they move on between stages. This helps to give members a sense of control over what they are going through. It also helps to normalize their experience and symptoms. Yalom and Vinogradov (1988) speak about the "shoulds" of people and society, such as that one should grieve for a certain period of time or in a certain way. Members report family and friends telling them, "You shouldn't cry anymore," "You should be over it already," "You should start dating," and "You should throw away all those old cloths of his." Dismissing these "shoulds" helps individuals to move through the bereavement process at a pace that is right for them.

The group emphasizes that there is no time line to bereavement. My group members often tell new members not to listen to anyone who tells them they should be "over it" or be able to stop crying, and that bereaved individuals need to be sensitive to themselves and not compare their bereavement process to anyone else's. Often individuals are relieved to find that others are having the same difficulty they are and that they are not alone. Other educational issues that are discussed in group can range from ways to deal with insomnia to the pros and cons of anti-depressant or anti-anxiety medication.

Another advantage of group therapy for elderly bereavement as opposed to individual therapy is that it allows members to become emotionally involved with other members. When members are able to get out of themselves and reach out and help other members, by lending emotional support, saying "I feel that way too," or giving practical advice, it takes the focus off themselves and their problems and gives them a positive feeling for being able to help someone. The majority of people in the elderly bereavement groups tend to be women. Many of the women in my groups were caretakers for their families and spouses and got their sense of identity from this. This may have been emphasized even more strongly if they were taking care of their husband's medical needs in the end of his life. When this role ends they experience a loss of identity. Group has been therapeutic by allowing them to care for others in the group and learn that they can keep the identity of being a caretaker by helping others or doing volunteer work, even though it is not taking care of their husband.

Yalom and Vinogradov (1988) discuss how the loss of familiar roles and concerns about finding a new identity affect the bereaved and this was also evident in my groups. Having to relinquish old roles leads to feelings of helplessness and inadequacy because some of the very things that defined a person's identity have disappeared or changed. A search for a new identity and a new meaning in life become important themes. Many group members had families with traditional roles. The females were the caretakers. They cooked, cleaned, did laundry, and were in charge of the social planning. The males handled the finances, did the driving, and handled all of the mechanical and repair work. When the spouse dies, the bereaved have to find ways to learn the roles that their spouse used to perform in order to survive. Group members encourage each other to try on these new roles and send the message that one might have learned much more about how to perform their spouse's role through living with them than they are aware.

With the loss of one's role in life comes the search for a new meaning to life and the search for ways to enjoy life even without their spouse being present. Group members often speak of how moving on and enjoying life does not mean that one is forgetting their spouse. Often, however, before members can start enjoying life again they need to deal with issues of guilt for enjoying life while their spouse is not there to share it with them. In the early phases members report feeling guilty for everything from laughing to eating the food their spouse liked or even for being alive. One group member who struggled with this issue for a long time returned to group after going on a cruise to report how freeing it felt to be able to enjoy herself without feeling guilty. She let herself have her moments of sadness at the start of the cruise that her husband was not there with her and let her tears out but then went on and enjoyed herself. Some group members allow themselves to start having new experiences that they did not have while their spouse was around. They start taking classes, join different types of community or social groups, learn new hobbies such as making jewelry or writing poetry, or start doing volunteer work. One group member got a job packing groceries and pushing the carts out to cars and found it to be a wonderful social opportunity. He cherished the ability to spend the day with people socializing and being involved with life again.

Group provides new opportunities for socialization, making friends, and developing a support network. I often encourage group members to exchange phone numbers with each other to get them interacting outside of the group. They then know there is someone they can call for support when they are having a bad day or night or just need someone with whom to talk. Most suffer from loneliness so just having someone to meet for lunch once a week and getting the individual out of the house can be a major accomplishment. Another wonderful thing I have seen in the group is more advanced members calling others members and giving them support and getting them out of the house. Not only does this benefit the less advanced member, it also benefits the member who is doing the giving. Around the time of anniversaries, birthdays, and holidays, group members have expressed how helpful it was to have other members calling to check on them and offer support and how it helped them to feel they were not alone in their grief.

The issue of bereavement in the elderly seems to be ideally suited to a group therapy approach. While individual therapy can be very helpful, the group can provide many things that are therapeutic to the individual which are not usually available in individual therapy. These curative factors include strong social support by peers and an avenue for socialization that can decrease feelings of isolation, an opportunity to get out of one's self and help others in the group, acceptance and normalization of one's grieving process by peers who can relate, the potential to be able to deal with strong and painful affect with individuals who have shared the same experience, the instillation of hope through the observation of more advanced group members and the opportunity to see that with time the pain will decrease and enjoyment in life can be found, the opportunity to learn new roles and skills, and a new opportunity for self-expression. In an age where the elderly population is continually increasing, it is important for therapists to know not only that group therapy is a cost and time efficient method of treatment, but that it is also a very effective treatment modality for the elderly who are suffering from bereavement.

REFERENCES

Roy, P. & Sumpter, H. (1983). Group support for the recently bereaved. *Health and Social Work, 8*(3), 230-232.

Sanders, Catherine (1989). Grief, the mourning after. New York: John Wiley and Sons.

Silverman, P., MacKenzie, D., Pellipas, M., & Wilson, E., eds. (1974). Helping each other in widowhood. New York: Health Sciences.

Yalom, Irvin D. (1975). The theory and practice of group psychotherapy (2nd ed.) New York: Basic Books, Inc.

Yalom, Irvin D. & Vinogradov, Sophia (1988). Bereavement Groups: techniques and themes. *International Journal of Group Psychotherapy, 38*(4), 419-445.

Group Psychotherapy and Group Work in Israel–1998

Haim Weinberg

SUMMARY. Israelis have a reputation for being quite individualistic, but no one can compete with their social and group spirit. This quality is prominent especially in times of personal and national distress. The public's quest for mutual help and affiliation needs are especially apparent during these stressful periods. When an Israeli is in distress, friends, neighbors, and good people will surround him to offer material or spiritual assistance. When the nation experiences difficulties, such as periods of war or waves of terror attacks, there are many spontaneous expressions of mutual help, cohesion, and getting together. There is an interesting phenomenon in Israel; group therapy blossoms after each war. People become interested in group work and more therapeutic

Haim Weinberg, MA, has degrees in Electronic Engineering, Psychology and Clinical Psychology. He is on faculty of the Tel-Aviv University where he teaches in the group-leader's training program within the school of social work. He also teaches group therapy at Beit-Berl college. Mr. Weinberg supervises clinicians in group therapy and has been in private practice for over twenty years. He is president of the Israeli Association of Group Psychotherapy and forum leader for the five hundred international members of the American Psychological Association Group Psychotherapy Listserv over the Internet. Mr. Weinberg is an international lecturer in the specialty of group psychotherapy and has chaired many conferences in Israel which focus on the efficacy of group psychotherapy. He has been published in many journals and his publishings have included such topics as Group Psychotherapy, Narcissistic and Borderline Couples, Trauma and Recovery, and Dynamic Approaches to Couple Therapy. He is both a member of the International Association of Group Psychotherapy and the American Group Psychotherapy Association.

The author gratefully acknowledges editorial assistance from Judith Simon, MSW.

[Haworth co-indexing entry note]: "Group Psychotherapy and Group Work in Israel–1998." Weinberg, Haim. Co-published simultaneously in *Journal of Psychotherapy in Independent Practice* (The Haworth Press, Inc.) Vol. 1, No. 2, 2000, pp. 43-51; and: *Group Therapy in Independent Practice* (ed: Scott Simon Fehr) The Haworth Press, Inc., 2000, pp. 43-51. Single or multiple copies of this article are available for a fee from The Haworth Document Delivery Service [1-800-342-9678, 9:00 a.m.–5:00 p.m. (EST). E-mail address: getinfo@haworthpressinc.com].

43

groups become available. *[Article copies available for a fee from The Haworth Document Delivery Service: 1-800-342-9678. E-mail address: getinfo@haworthpressinc.com <Website: http://www.haworthpressinc.com>]*

KEYWORDS. Group psychotherapy, Israel

THE CURRENT SITUATION OF GROUP THERAPY AND GROUP-WORK IN ISRAEL

Prior to 1994 there was scant attention to the group modality. Group psychotherapy has garnered greater interest and attention in the last few years following the national group therapy conference that year. The keynote speakers were Irvin Yalom (on his first visit to Israel) and Earl Hopper. These world-renowned experts contributed to the success of this conference. The signs of group therapy's development are numerous and are prominent in many dimensions: A growth in the number of therapists who are engaged in group-work, a rise in the number and variety of groups taking place (especially in the areas of social work), a sharp increase in the number of newly available group leaders' training programs and in the number of students in training. Several outstanding group-psychotherapists from abroad came to Israel lately for seminars, conferences or workshops (among them Irvin Yalom, Earl Hopper, Malcolm Pines, Roy MacKenzie, Walter Stone, Morris Nitsun). On the other hand, more Israelis present papers and workshops in international conferences of group-therapy (in the last conference of the International Association of Group-Psychotherapy in London, August 98, there were 22 presentations by Israelis). The Institute of Group Analysis (IGA) from London opened a training course in group-analysis in Israel for senior therapists. The last two years, 1996-98, has seen an increase in the number of conferences and seminars in the field of group work and group therapy and a doubling of the number of members in the Israeli Association of Group Psychotherapy. A deficiency persists in the availability of Hebrew language books (either original or translated). Fluency in English allows access to the original books; others must be limited to older books and few anthologies.

Group psychotherapy in Israel is primarily influenced by the British schools of thought. American clinicians and theoreticians are less well known. The leading and most valued scholar is Wilfred Bion. The work of Foulkes is becoming increasingly respected. Beside Yalom (following his recent visit to Israel), American clinicians and writers are unknown in Israel. In groups that are not "task focused," the orientation is psychodynamic. On the other hand, the behavioral model influences the practical group work done by social workers in public welfare services (e.g., domestic violence, children of divorce, wives of the chronically ill). These specific groups are generally not psychodynamic.

GROUP LEADERS' TRAINING IN ISRAEL

While group therapists in Israel maintain a high standard in their work, most group leaders are engaged in this area as secondary to their individual therapy work and do not define themselves as group psychotherapists. In Israel there is no official certification for group therapists such as the Certified Group Psychotherapist (CGP) in America. Anyone can lead a group; certification as a psychotherapist is not mandatory. The primary therapeutic training is for individual work. Psychologists, psychiatrists, and social workers that would like to work in this area usually learn it through "on the job training" and mostly because of managers' coercion. Those who do want to learn it in a systematic way can enroll in diploma courses that are usually associated with university social work departments. The basic requirements for acceptance are an acknowledged certification in psychotherapy and some experience in individual work. The number of applicants to these programs outnumbers the number of possible students, making this a highly selective process. Group training programs in Israel usually combine studies of one day per week for two years. However, there is no program exclusively dedicated to group-psychotherapy. If we compare the studies in these programs to the Faculty core course manual published by the AGPA (American Group Psychotherapy Association) we will find that the studies in Israel are more intensive. For example, instead of a 12 hours' introductory course required for the CGP by AGPA, the theoretical course in the group leaders' training programs in Israel lasts a full semester (28 hours). In addition, the students participate in a sensitivity group for one semester, take a specific course on group leader's skills, watch a live group behind a one-way mirror, co-lead a group with a senior group-leader and are supervised for their leading.

WHO ARE THE GROUP LEADERS IN ISRAEL?

As mentioned before, every one can be a group leader in Israel, but usually group therapy is led by psychotherapeutic experts such as psychiatrists, psychologists, social workers and expressive therapists (art, movement, music, etc.). Although there is not yet an alphabetical index or data base of group therapists in Israel, we can get an idea about who is doing group work in Israel by analyzing the professional distribution of the Israel Association of Group Psychotherapy members. As can be seen from the table, about one third of the group psychotherapists are psychologists (almost three quarters of them are clinical psychologists), and almost 30% are social workers. Overall, a variety of experts in the therapeutic/counseling professions are doing group therapy in Israel. The number of those leading groups after graduating from training programs is increasing.

TYPICAL ISSUES ON GROUP WORK IN ISRAEL

Most of the work done in Israeli groups is similar to what can be seen in any other place in the world, and the subjects dealt with are

TABLE 1. Professions distribution of the IAGP members (May 98)

Percentage	Number	Profession
25.9%	64	Clinical Psychologist
8.9%	22	Other Psychologist
29.6%	73	Social Worker
4.9%	12	Psychiatrist
8.9%	22	Expressive Therapist
4.9%	12	Educational Counselor
3.6%	9	Organization Counselor
1.2%	3	Family Therapist
12.1%	30	Other
100%	247	Total

universal. But, there are some unique issues that face groups in Israel. These subjects can arise in therapeutic groups, or be elaborated thoroughly in specific subject groups: conflict groups (Arab-Jews relations, left-right politics, and religious non-religious) second generation of Holocaust survivors, PTSD and reactions to wars and terrorists' attacks. There is a lot of investment in social integration and post-traumatic issues. For example, these are some of the works presented in the Israeli group-psychotherapy conference in December 1997: (1) The division between "us" and "them"–as a universal social structure; (2) A journey of a Jewish-Arabic group–between personal and group processes, (3) Loss and bereavement in the experience of the group-therapist, (4) The open and concealed social identity (ethnic, national, gender) in the group process, (5) Groups in social-cultural conflict, (6) Parallel processes in the joint space of widows and orphans' group, vs. the co-leaders' unit, (7) Groups for adolescents' parents in bereaved families, (8) A journey to the past–Holocaust child survivors deal with their memories through autobiographic writing group, (9) Couple group for second generation of Holocaust survivors, (10) Group intervention with survivors of a terror attack through CISD (critical incident stress debriefing), (11) Combined individual and group intervention with survivors of a terrorist attack.

Times of war, waves of terrorist threats and periods of military insecurity become manifest in the group; the intense atmosphere might be reflected in acted-out aggression or expressed through subjects of existential anxieties raised in the group. Sometimes the group-leader can identify parallel process between what is going on in the group and in society at large, as defense mechanisms of split and projective identification are very intensive. The group may find a scapegoat and attack him/her with cruelty, or identify sub-groups as enemies and fight them.

In situations like these the group leaders deal with a complicated and difficult countertransference, because the emotional and psychological processes in the group challenge the leader's ability to maintain an objective viewpoint. This can happen either because of the intensity or the fact that the leaders are also involved with these sociological processes.

These situations make it difficult for the group-leaders to secure the group boundaries and remain sensitive to the inner worlds of the participant and/or the whole group. The threatening reality enters the group forcefully through its contents and dynamics. For example: after a terror attack with many casualties, the group was talking about what happened. Although the group therapist thought that this conversation was related to the aggression in the group, it was hard for him to say anything about it. Another vivid example followed the assassination of the Israeli Prime Minister Rabin. Only a non-Israeli group therapist could interpret the discussion in the group about the event as unconsciously expressing a wish or fear from exterminating the group leader. A very clear example of this difficulty was the situation in Israel during the Gulf War (1991). Citizens had to remain in sealed rooms, fearing a gas attack from Iraq. The group therapists that tried to continue groups in sealed rooms were sharing the same anxiety, distress and uncertainty as the group participants.

UNIQUE PHENOMENA IN THE GROUP PROCESS

Compared to other countries, the level of interpersonal tolerance in the beginning of an Israeli group is quite low, and the level of aggression is quite high. Actually this phenomenon is correlated with some psychological aspects typical of Israeli society: Israelis tend to express aggression when they feel vulnerable. Hiding weakness and presenting apparent strength is the cultural norm. This may be a result of the need to be different from the Jew from the Diaspora who is perceived as weak and therefore chased. It is clear that years of living in a country surrounded by enemies enforced the need not to reveal any signs of weakness. In the group, expressions of anger replace vulnerability or pain, and group therapists must be empathic to this.

Another typical characteristic of life in Israel is permanent intrusion and breaking personal boundaries. Practically this can be expressed in insensitive comments that impinge privacy (such as commenting about the other's look or dress) or with personal questions that in any other place in the world would seem rude. It takes a long time for a group to learn to give effective and unoffending feedback and to show interest in others with real care and empathy.

Another aspect of boundaries is the Israeli tendency to break any rule, test the limits, and reject authority. The Israelis do not like being told what to do. The group contract, e.g., time limits, can be a serious obstacle to the group work. In contrast to the US, where the participants usually collaborate and cooperate with authority, an Israeli's initial reaction is to test the limits. Being on time is a rare phenomenon; coming late to the group is typical. There are other countries where it may be difficult to start the group on time, e.g., in South America, where there are different societal norms regarding time.

SPECIAL POPULATIONS IN ISRAEL

People who grew up in the kibbutz are one of the special populations. The influence of the kibbutzim on the Israeli society and the national ethos is greater than would be expected by the small percentage of the kibbutz members in the general population. The kibbutz-born are regarded as the elite of the Israeli society. A large proportion of them volunteer to serve in the special-best units of the Israeli Defence Force or become officers in the army. Usually, the kibbutz-born are very conforming and are easily influenced by social pressure. The kibbutz experience is a group experience. When students who come to study group work are asked about their first memory of a group, there are always some people who would say "all my life I remember myself in a group." These are the kibbutz-born. They live in a group from birth, are toilet trained together, eat in a group, take showers together, and in the past they also slept together in the "children-house" and not with their parents. These facts largely influence their personality and relation to the group. Along with the many advantages that growing up in a group has, there are also many disadvantages, especially being quite conformist, yielding to social consensus and having difficulty expressing their individuality.

One's personal history of early group experiences and one's experience of the family of origin accompanies a new group member. For "kibbutz graduates," the experience is always associated with the primary kibbutz group and usually the associations are negative. "Kibbutz refugees" are usually deterred from joining a therapeutic group because for them, who are coming from a culture of conformity and yielding to group pressure, the group is perceived as freedom-robbing and not as enhancing personal space.

Another population frequently met in therapeutic groups is the second generation of Holocaust survivors. Much has been written about this population and its specific characteristics. As mentioned before, there are special groups for Holocaust survivors and their offspring as well as specific organizations that offer psychological services solely for this population. Unique behavior patterns typical of this population are evident in the developing relationships in the group. One sees great sensitivity to guilt feelings and a tendency to take upon oneself excessive guilt or react with anger to criticism, over-protection in relation to others in the group and excessive sensitivity to the others' needs while not listening to the needs of the self. Additionally, one observes difficulty in dealing with aggression and self-assertion. All these and others are salient in the group. Working through them in the "here and now" and connecting them to their sources can help to effect changes in these interpersonal patterns.

Israeli society is a "melting pot," integrating immigrants from all over the world. Although the major immigrations have ended and the proportion of the Israeli-born is growing, it is not rare to find people who were born in Argentina, the former USSR or the US in one therapy group. It is common to have patients whose parents emigrated from diverse locations, e.g., Eastern and Western Europe, Asia and Africa. This phenomenon creates a rich and colorful texture in describing the background of each of the group members. In the same group you can hear about Polish parents who seed guilt feelings in their children and about Moroccan parents who emotionally tie their children through the tribal enmeshment of the extended family. Initially, the group members may sound very different from one another, as everyone comes from a different background with very different norms and cultural values. In addition, as it happens in society at large, it may create status differences and stereotypes or judgmental evaluation of people from different origins. The task of the group-leader is to help the group members to bridge the gaps and find the similarities between different congregations without relinquishing the uniqueness of each participant.

CONCLUSION

In this article I tried to describe group psychotherapy and group work in Israel. Group leading in Israel has some unique features frequently expressed in the subjects addressed in the group (Holocaust, terror and social conflicts), typical populations (kibbutz born, second generation of Holocaust survivors, and immigrants from different nations), and in typical Israeli dynamics (expressions of aggression and criticism, intrusion and difficulty with boundaries).

Group work in Israel has been growing and expanding in recent years. Although the training of group therapists in Israel is kept on high standards and there are quality group psychotherapists, little is known of this work outside Israel.

It is my hope that this article serves as an introduction to the group therapy work that we are doing in Israel as well as contributing to an understanding of our unique cultural challenges as they relate to psychotherapy. As worldwide communication expands, cross-pollination of ideas and experiences enriches clinicians of all nationalities and persuasions.

The Role of Group Therapy in Promoting Identity Development in ADHD Adolescents

David Cantor

SUMMARY. This paper examines the role that group psychotherapy plays in promoting the development of identity in adolescents who are diagnosed with Attention Deficit Disorder with Hyperactivity (ADHD). Negotiating identity issues is the central task of adolescence (Erikson, 1950). It is also one of the most difficult periods for ADHD adolescents because of their innate and learned sensitivities to the experience of shame. Shame is the feeling we have when we evaluate ourselves using the standards of valued others and of society and determine that we do not meet those standards (Lewis, 1992). Group psychotherapy thus becomes the treatment of choice for adolescents diagnosed with ADHD because the process of group psychotherapy addresses the issues of identity and shame in a way that individual therapy is unable. *[Article copies available for a fee from The Haworth Document Delivery Service: 1-800-342-9678. E-mail address: getinfo@haworthpressinc.com <Website: http:// www.haworthpressinc.com>]*

KEYWORDS. Adolescents, group psychotherapy, ADHD, identity development

Dr. Cantor is Director of the Diagnostic Learning Center and Family Counseling Center in Kingsport, Tennessee. His clinical work focuses on the assessment of children and adults as well as providing individual, family, and group therapy. Dr. Cantor serves as Internship Supervisor and is on the Adjunct Faculty at East Tennessee State University. He trained at the Louisiana State University Medical School in New Orleans.

[Haworth co-indexing entry note]: "The Role of Group Therapy in Promoting Identity Development in ADHD Adolescents." Cantor, David. Co-published simultaneously in *Journal of Psychotherapy in Independent Practice* (The Haworth Press, Inc.) Vol. 1, No. 2, 2000, pp. 53-62; and: *Group Therapy in Independent Practice* (ed: Scott Simon Fehr) The Haworth Press, Inc., 2000, pp. 53-62. Single or multiple copies of this article are available for a fee from The Haworth Document Delivery Service [1-800-342-9678, 9:00 a.m. - 5:00 p.m. (EST). E-mail address: getinfo@haworthpressinc.com].

INTRODUCTION

This paper examines the role that group psychotherapy plays in promoting the development of identity in adolescents who are diagnosed with Attention Deficit Disorder with Hyperactivity (ADHD). The core symptoms of ADHD include hyperactivity, impulsivity, and inattention (DSM-IV, 1994). These symptoms must have been present before the age of seven and must manifest themselves in two or more settings. ADHD currently affects approximately 3 to 7% of all school-age children and adolescents (Barkley, 1997).

In addition, adolescents who are diagnosed with ADHD often develop other emotional difficulties. Externalizing disorders such as Oppositional Defiant Disorder and Conduct Disorder are the most common while Depression is the most common type of internalizing disorder. The externalizing co-morbidities are the most common because children and adolescents with ADHD prefer to focus on or act on the world rather than to focus on themselves and be reacted upon. Shame plays a major role in why this is so.

Negotiating identity issues is the central task of adolescence (Erikson, 1950). It is their time of finding out who they are and what they believe. This is a time of self-definition for the adolescent as well as a time of owning and disowning (McConville, 1995). It also is a time of moving into the social world of others and moving away from the family structure, which tends to create anxieties for the adolescent and their families.

The period of identity development is one of the most difficult periods for ADHD adolescents because of their innate and learned sensitivities to the experience of shame. The essential features in sensitivity to shame and its emotional variants, embarrassment, humiliation, and mortification, are the wish not to know and the wish not to see or be seen. Resolution of identity issues requires seeing and knowing oneself while also allowing oneself to be seen and known by others emotionally.

Group psychotherapy thus becomes the treatment of choice for ADHD adolescents. This is because the process of group therapy operates in the arena of emotional self-disclosure by the group members. Emotional self-disclosure by the adolescent facilitates the process of seeing and knowing both intrapersonally and interpersonally. It is this seeing and knowing which promotes identity development in ADHD adolescents. In addition, group psychotherapy emphasizes the successful resolution of the identity crisis by means of a positive peer group affiliation (Rachman, 1975).

The above thesis is not to discount the value of medications such as Ritalin and Adderall, nor the value of individual psychotherapy. Medication therapy, though often helpful and frequently recommended, is generally not sufficient to address all the ADHD adolescent's needs. Individual psychotherapy, while being useful for developing initial rapport and for addressing treatment management issues, does not reach the heart of the matter when dealing with ADHD adolescents. At the heart of the matter is adolescent identity development.

Erik Erikson (1950) has taught us succinctly the importance of identity development in the adolescent's emotional world. When the process of identity development is going along smoothly, the adolescent can experience a sense of confidence and security. However, when this process becomes conflictual and bumpy, the adolescent experiences a wide range of feelings including shame, anxiety, anger or rage, and insecurity. The adolescent who is experiencing the developmental stage of an identity crisis alternates between the experiences of ego identity and identity confusion.

The search for ego identity and the frequently associated identity confusion are seen in group by the different roles with which the adolescent will experiment. For example, one young female adolescent in group could not make up her mind as to which clique she best belonged. During one particular group she expressed feelings that she was a "redneck party" girl and then switched to talking about how well she fit in with the "preppies" and then later in the group discussed how she took pride in her sports abilities and how she seemed to fit in with the "jocks." The group therapist and the group members helped her to see that her identity could incorporate all these supposedly different ways of being into one identity. She learned over time that identity is made up of various facets and ways of being.

The search for ego identity is also seen in the topics brought up for group discussion by the ADHD adolescent. Levy-Warren (1996) writes that adolescents are often focused on issues of sameness and differentness in themselves, their families, and their friends. These issues can be explicitly explored in group therapy in a way that cannot be matched in individual psychotherapy.

Many of the discussions that take place in an ADHD adolescent group center around the commonalities and differences that they share. In the beginning these discussions stay somewhat superficial and are focused on matters like school affiliation and common recreational interests. As the group develops and matures, the discussions then become centered around emotional similarities and differences in areas such as beliefs, values, and emotional reactions to criticism, rejection, and embarrassment.

Rachman (1975) writes that adolescents must develop peer group affiliation to ego identity. Group therapy provides adolescents with the opportunity to gain this crucial peer group affiliation in a way that is fostering of identity and emotional growth. Rachman (1975) writes that the group psychotherapist must serve as an identity role model for the adolescent group. He or she must function as an active, emotionally involved, positive adult authority who fosters a beneficial relationship with the adolescents. The therapist does this with honest and judicious self-disclosure along with curiosity toward all the thoughts and feelings that are expressed in the group session. This is effective because ADHD adolescents are used to adults who foreclose any exploration with advice on what the adolescent ought to do and how they ought to behave.

One young man was particularly affected by the fact that the group was not about going around the group telling each other what to do. It was more about learning about oneself, one's feelings, and one's ways of interacting with others that was separate from the diagnosis or label that he carried. He told the group that he thought our time would be spent learning things specifically aimed at helping him in school and with his hyperactivity. One astute group member responded to him that what the group was about was learning about your feelings and your beliefs and it did not matter if you had ADHD or not. This captured the essence of what ADHD adolescent groups should be about. These groups should leave diagnoses at the door and instead focus on the issues of identity development.

Ormont (1992) writes about several factors which are beneficial in the process of group psychotherapy. An important one for our discussion is the idea that group psychotherapy provides the opportunity for emotionally salient self-definition. He writes that the patient gets to find out how s/he looks, how s/he comes across to others, and the opportunity to discover what he or she actually feels when dealing with people. This process is extremely important for ADHD adolescents because of their tendency to act impulsively with others and also their tendency to not pay attention to their feelings and thoughts. When adolescents can practice the process of self-definition in group psychotherapy, it paves the way for more effective self-definition and identity formation outside of the group experience.

Adolescents with ADHD have a harder time developing a stable identity not only because of the genetic basis of their disorder but also because of the messages that they receive from their environment. Barkley (1997) writes that these children often receive more harsh judgments and punishments, moral denigration, and social rejection than other children. They are commonly seen as reckless, lazy, impulsive, selfish, unmotivated, thoughtless, immature, and irresponsible. This, of course, affects the ADHD person's feelings about him/herself and increases his/her feelings of shame.

Adolescents with ADHD frequently have grown up receiving the message that they are not good enough. This message is sent by both teachers and parents who see the adolescent as not living up to society's standards of academic and behavioral competence. Conformity is highly prized in our society and when a person marches to the "beat of a different drummer," s/he is often labeled as being inferior or less than. Children often internalize this message and use it to judge themselves. The resulting judgments produce a profound sense of shame.

One young man who participated in the ADHD adolescent group told how all through elementary and middle school he had been considered different by both his peers and his teachers because of his hyperactivity, short attention span, and impulsivity. He reported that he even had one teacher mock his hyperactivity in the classroom, to the class's amusement and to his humiliation. Unfortunately, his story is a very common example of how ADHD children are treated and how they respond with feelings of shame and lowered self-esteem.

Shame is the feeling we have when we evaluate ourselves using the standards of valued others and of society and determine that we do not meet those standards (Lewis, 1992). It produces within us the desire to hide from the judgmental gaze of others. It also involves a belief that there is something wrong with the self. Nathanson (1992) writes that shame seems to involve a sudden decrease in self-esteem related to a moment in which we are revealed to be somewhat less than we want to believe. Lee (1996) puts it into an interpersonal context by writing that shame is that cringe we feel when we discover or imagine that the connection we desire is threatened in some way.

Shame is not easily processed or consciously examined by adolescents and especially not by adolescents who tend to have difficulties with impulsivity and with attention and concentration. Lewis (1971) writes very succinctly about the phenomenon of by-passed shame. By-passed shame occurs when the individual is unable to process the feelings of shame and instead substitutes another feeling in its place. The two most common feelings that are expressed instead of shame are rage and sadness. These experiences of rage and sadness, if not appropriately responded to, may become chronic and thus lead to Conduct disorder and/or Depression.

In an ADHD adolescent group, feelings of shame are often dealt with either by withdrawal or by playing the clown. At times when the topic of discussion, for example academics or sexuality, was one in which shame and embarrassment played a major part, the group would compete with each other in order to see who could be the funniest and the silliest. The best therapeutic response to situations like these is to allow the tension to be discharged via humor and then to invite two of the group members to begin a dialogue about the subject matter. This is done by having one group member question another group member regarding his feelings about the topic. By creating a dialogue between members, a bridge is built both interpersonally between members and also between the group member and his own feelings (Ormont, 1996).

Shame is also commonly defended against through the use of the defense mechanism of projection. Projection is a common defense mechanism of adolescence. McConville (1995) writes that teenagers have a remarkable capacity for projecting unwanted aspects of themselves and seeing themselves as victims and making others responsible for the outcomes of their own behavior. ADHD adolescents in particular tend to use this defense frequently when dealing with other adolescents.

One goal in group therapy with ADHD adolescents which is related to shame and projection is to help the young person reclaim or reown aspects of himself which are frequently and impulsively projected onto others. This must be done gently and in the context of a positive therapeutic alliance due to the shame-sensitivity that the ADHD adolescent frequently experiences. In addition, it is helpful when the group members are able to confront each other on the aspects which are projected. Frequently, adolescents can have a better sense of what another adolescent is projecting than can an adult therapist. Finally, when the group environment is a positive one, messages from the ADHD adolescent's peers are often heard more clearly than messages received from an adult.

Morrel (1998) writes that feelings are the core of subjectivity and the royal road to self-knowledge. Self-knowledge is the royal road to resolving the developmental task of identity consolidation. Thus, the goal of group therapy is to enable the ADHD adolescent to experience his full range of feelings without needing to either act on them immediately or to deny them. Curiosity on the part of the group therapist and on the part of the ADHD adolescent can make that an achievable goal.

Wexler (1991) writes that the most important goal of therapy is to help adolescents learn to identify and label internal states. He writes that it is important for them to be able to use feelings as a form of self-signaling rather than as a trigger for reacting impulsively. This is especially true for ADHD adolescents who tend to react impulsively when presented with emotional stimuli. In an ADHD group, it is important for the therapist and the members as a team to focus on and pay attention to all the feelings, including those that are not directly expressed.

Universality (Yalom, 1975) is an important factor in the effectiveness of group therapy for ADHD adolescents. This is because it directly confronts the feelings of shame about being different. Sharing feelings about taking medication and the disappointments often experienced in both the academic and interpersonal arenas help create a group culture of acceptance and non-judgmentalness. When the ADHD adolescent can come to terms with the fact that difference does not make inferiority, his self-esteem and handling of other emotional issues becomes enhanced.

There are two additional group processes which are considered to be effective and need to be nurtured in group psychotherapy with ADHD adolescents. These processes fall under the rubric of Yalom's (1975) ideas about the value of interpersonal learning.

The first process observed is the group therapist's interaction as an authority figure with each unique individual in the group. By observing an interaction that is happening outside the self but still related to issues closely related to the self, the adolescent is able to process the issues and feelings more effectively and gain insight into both others and himself. One way to make observed processes real to each group member is to go around the group and ask each group member what he feels about the interaction that was observed.

The second process observed is the handling of emotions by the group therapist within a social or interpersonal setting. It is a much more powerful experience for the adolescent to observe his group therapist handling an emotion such as anger in an interpersonal or in vivo situation than just to hear the therapist explain the principles of how to handle an emotionally charged situation. After utilizing appropriate self-disclosure, it is important to invite the group to comment on their feelings about what has been occurring. The goal is to get them paying attention to their feelings and then talking about them. It is this process of paying attention to feelings and then communicating them in an interpersonal setting that promotes identity development.

The group psychotherapist in ADHD groups should also pay very close attention to his/her own feelings. Ormont (1992) writes that the therapist who doesn't know what he's feeling will err in understanding, in interpretation, in timing–in all aspects of technique. This is especially true in ADHD groups because of the profound need ADHD adolescents have of a positive adult figure who can teach them the value of being in touch with the emotional aspects of their personalities. This is also true because being able to reflect on one's feelings provides the necessary emotional space in which to delay one's impulses or reactions. Thus emotional reflection becomes an important ally in dealing with impulsivity, one of the core symptoms of ADHD.

A factor which is important to our discussion is that group psychotherapy yields on-the-spot experience (Ormont, 1992). This is congruent with Yalom's (1975) idea of the importance of emphasizing the here-and-now in group discussions. ADHD adolescents need the experience of being able to ask themselves and to be asked what they are feeling as an interpersonal scenario is being played out. The reason that this is important is because the identification and labeling of feelings and attitudes forms the bedrock for identity development. The identification and labeling of one's own feelings as well as sensitivity to other's feelings is the actual process of interpersonal knowing which is crucial for a successful identity stage resolution.

CONCLUSION

This article has examined the role that group psychotherapy plays in promoting the development of identity in ADHD adolescents. Negotiating the identity developmental crisis is the primary task of adolescence. It is also a task in which ADHD adolescents have more difficulty. Shame and especially shame which is by-passed is a primary impediment along the path of identity resolution. Group therapy in order to be effective with ADHD adolescents must address the issues of identity development and by-passed shame. Each adolescent in the group must have the chance to explore who s/he is and what s/he believes in an environment of acceptance without judgment. It is the group therapist, through being an identity role model, who initially creates this type of environment. Optimally, the group members then will take on this role and begin to create it for themselves both inside the group and outside the group via internalization of group processes.

REFERENCES

American Psychiatric Association. (1994). Diagnostic and statistical manual of mental disorders (4th ed.). Washington, DC: Author.

Barkley, R. A. (1997). ADHD and the nature of self-control. New York: Guilford Press.

Erikson, E. H. (1950, 1963). Childhood and society, 2nd edition. New York: W.W. Norton & Company.

Lee, R. G. (1996). Shame and the gestalt model. In Robert G. Lee and Gordon Wheeler (Eds.) The voice of shame: Silence and connection in psychotherapy. San Francisco: Jossey-Bass Publishers.

Levy-Warren, M. (1996). The adolescent journey: development, identity formation, and psychotherapy. Northvale, NJ: Jason Aronson.

Lewis, H. B. (1971). Shame and guilt in neurosis. New York: International Universities Press.

Lewis, M. (1992). Shame: the exposed self. New York: The Free Press.

McConville, M. (1995). Adolescence: psychotherapy and the emergent self. San Francisco: Jossey Bass Publishers.

Morrel, A. (1998). Attention Deficit Disorder and Its Relationship to Narcissistic Pathology. In P. Beren (Ed.). Narcissistic Disorders in Children and Adolescents: Diagnosis and Treatment. North Vale. New Jersey: Jason Aronson, Inc.

Nathanson, D. L. (1992). Shame and pride: affect, sex, and the birth of the self. New York: W.W. Norton & Company.

Ormont, L. (1992). The group therapy experience: from theory to practice. New York: St. Martin's Press.

Rachman, A. (1975). Identity group psychotherapy with adolescents. Northvale, NJ: Jason Aronson.

Wexler, D. (1991). The adolescent self: strategies for self-management, self-soothing, and self-esteem in Adolescents. New York: W.W. Norton & Company.

Yalom, I. (1975). The theory and practice of group psychotherapy. 2nd Edition. New York: Basic Books.

Anger in Group Therapy, Countertransference and the Novice Group Therapist

Steven L. Van Wagoner

SUMMARY. Although no therapist likes to be the object of intense anger in groups, group therapists in training particularly struggle with how to therapeutically deal with its expression, especially as it produces strong countertransference reactions, interferes with their expectations to be helpful and compassionate, and threatens their self-esteem with feelings of shame and failure. Broadening the definition of countertransference to include both objective, or realistic elements of the therapist's reactions to the personality of the patient, as well as the subjective elements stemming from the therapist's own neurotic and narcissistic needs, offers supervisors a broader framework and repertoire of techniques for aiding supervisees in the exploration of countertransference. Thus the supervisory focus can be on countertransference exploration as both a potential impediment to treatment, as well as a powerful tool for furthering the therapeutic work in group. The advantages and dilemmas inherent in supervisor and supervisee participation as co-therapists in a psychotherapy group are discussed. *[Article copies available for a fee from The Haworth Document Delivery Service: 1-800-342-9678. E-mail address: getinfo@haworthpressinc.com <Website: http://www.haworthpressinc.com>]*

KEYWORDS. Group psychotherapy, countertransference, clinical training

---

Dr. Van Wagoner is the Coordinator of Group Therapy at The George Washington University Counseling Center. He is also an Adjunct Assistant Professor in the Clinical Psychology Program at The George Washington University and Adjunct Assistant Professor in the Counseling Psychology Program at the University of Maryland. Dr. Van Wagoner has been published in the areas of group and individual psychotherapy in a number of journals and books. He maintains an active private practice in Washington, DC and has been running groups for the past 16 years.

[Haworth co-indexing entry note]: "Anger in Group Therapy, Countertransference and the Novice Group Therapist." Van Wagoner, Steven L. Co-published simultaneously in *Journal of Psychotherapy in Independent Practice* (The Haworth Press, Inc.) Vol. 1, No. 2, 2000, pp. 63-75; and: *Group Therapy in Independent Practice* (ed: Scott Simon Fehr) The Haworth Press, Inc., 2000, pp. 63-75. Single or multiple copies of this article are available for a fee from The Haworth Document Delivery Service [1-800-342-9678, 9:00 a.m. - 5:00 p.m. (EST). E-mail address: getinfo@haworthpressinc.com].

INTRODUCTION

Therapy groups, by nature of multiple positive, negative, and ambivalent transference relationships contain both pervasive anxiety and aggression that are inevitable byproducts of this confluence of individuals simultaneously seeking relief from discomfort and dysfunction in their lives and relationships (Slavson, 1957). At the center of the emotional exchange is the group therapist. It is in her that members harbor some hope for salvation from what ails them, but also extreme ambivalence about whether to accede this much authority to the leader. Many theorists propose that this ambivalence will build to a crescendo as authority issues are reenacted with the therapist and the other members, and that this build-up in tension and aggression characterizes general developmental sequences in the life of any group (Agazarian, 1994; Bennis & Shepard, 1956; Yalom, 1975). Whether or not one subscribes to the notion of a predictable sequence of group development, aggression is an inevitable aspect of all groups and when ignored or mishandled can obstruct therapeutic progress (Ormont, 1984).

In an ongoing therapy group consisting of undergraduate and graduate college students, Mary had been confronting Sol and Ed about what she perceived to be their ongoing tendency to monopolize sessions. She blamed them for forming their own sub-group at the exclusion of others, and accused them of being more concerned with their "social relationship" than what they could learn from each other and the rest of the group about the nature of their interpersonal problems. Mary was in emotional contact with the two men, and their discomfort, apparent by their pleading glances toward the therapists (an experienced group therapist and a doctoral intern in psychology), was a byproduct of this emotional exchange. While Sol seemed more anxious, as if wanting to flee, Ed appeared to be experiencing something wholly different. His face was flush, the muscles in his jaw tensed, and although the frequency of his glances toward the therapists rivaled Sol, the emotion appeared to be an intensifying anger. Mary, as if sensing this, suddenly turned on the senior therapist and railed, "Are you just going to sit there? This group is supposed to be helping me, and the only thing I feel like doing now is leaving. You're not helping them or me, and I feel like I'm the only one taking any responsibility in here right now! At least she (nods toward the trainee) has an excuse because she is new at this, but you should definitely be doing something more."

Depending upon the group dynamics in this particular group, the individual histories of the members, the length of time the group has been together, the theoretical orientation of the leader(s) and other factors, the therapist might attempt any number of interventions not limited to bridging (Ormont, 1990; 1997), an object oriented question (Spotnitz, 1976), a group-as-a-whole intervention, functional subgrouping (Agazarian, 1996), or confrontation. But what of Mary's discharge of anger and Ed's barely contained experience of it? There are powerful emotions present in the above exchange that could be the product of "real" or "objective" components of the interaction, as well as projections and projective identifications. How the group therapist deals with these emotions in the group members is paramount to the group's development or failure, but equally important, how the therapist manages his own emotional reactions to these exchanges can also greatly impact his effectiveness in the center of this emotional turmoil. While all therapists, experienced and neophyte, cannot help but be affected by emotionally intense communication between members, or members and themselves, for the beginning therapist this challenge is compounded by the experience of learning new skills, feelings of inadequacy, and the wish to be viewed as competent (Fosshage, 1997; Jacobs, David, & Meyer, 1995). A critical difference between the new group therapist and the experienced one, aside from a greater repertoire of skills, is that the experienced therapist often has a greater appreciation for the need to recognize, identify, and resolve countertransference reactions as a regular activity in the treatment of his patients. This is true of the myriad of emotions that are expressed in groups, but especially true of intense anger or seething rage. "Few experiences in the life of the mental health professional are more unpleasant than being intensely hated by a patient he is trying to help" (Gabbard, 1989).

It is beyond the scope of this paper to address all the potential transference-countertransference interactions group therapists can have with their group members and the group-as-a-whole. In this paper, therefore, I plan to examine potential therapist countertransference feelings in reaction to expression of anger in group therapy, since anger is an inevitable aspect of group development (Agazarian, 1996; Bennis & Shepard, 1956; Yalom, 1975), and in particular groups containing patients with preoedipal, narcissistic character disorders (Kirman, 1995; Spotnitz, 1976). I will attend less to issues pertaining to the clinical management of angry and aggressive feelings in groups (i.e., technique), examining instead the handling of countertransference reactions to its expression. Moreover, while group anger can place considerable strain on the most seasoned group therapist, the challenges it presents to the novice can be overwhelming. Many developing therapists fear their angry patients will leave group (Ormont, 1984); in addition, these fears can awaken primitive fears of abandonment (HarPaz, 1994) and shame (Hahn, 1995) in the therapist. Many leaders, and especially the novice, grasp for techniques that might restore some semblance of calm to the chaos that often accompanies aggressive communication in groups (Livingston & Livingston, 1998). Although quite understandable, it is the release and expression of aggression that is often critical to unblocking the barriers to maturational development that exist, particularly in the more narcissistically organized patient (Ormont, 1984; Spotnitz, 1976). Helping members unlock and express their aggressive feelings threatens to "destroy the [therapist's] capacities of sustaining, or recovering, his therapeutic intention toward the patient" (Epstein, 1979, p. 221). Therefore, contributing factors to this challenge for the novice, as well as recommendations for supervision will also be proposed.

COUNTERTRANSFERENCE

Classical psychoanalytic theory defines countertransference as those reactions to the patient's transference that are triggered by the analyst's own unconscious needs and neurotic conflicts, and therefore are to be identified, analyzed, and eliminated as potential contaminants to the therapeutic endeavor (Arlow, 1985; Freud, 1910/1959; Reich, 1951; 1960). Subsequent formulations about countertransference, however, have yielded a broader definition which would include all of the analyst's feelings and attitudes about the client, those stemming from the therapist's unconscious needs and conflicts, and those objective reactions to the patient that most people could be expected to have to a particular kind of patient (Fromm-Reichmann, 1950; Heiman, 1950; Kernberg, 1975). These latter theorists posit that countertransference can derail treatment if gone undetected or unanalyzed, but moreover they view these therapist reactions as a potential window to greater understanding of the patient since they provide important data about the interaction between therapist and client (Blanck & Blanck, 1979; Gelso & Carter, 1985; Peabody & Gelso, 1982). Countertransference reactions have the potential to provide the same important data about patients in group therapy, however, the reactions are typically more complicated and powerful than in individual therapy (Spotnitz, 1976); occur in response to multiple transference relationships (Grotjahn, 1953); and can stimulate powerful counterresistance to the group resistance (Rosenthal, 1987). Groups are often more likely to detect and address therapist countertransference, and provide considerable protection to members from therapist countertransference reactions (Rosenthal, 1987), thus contributing to heightened anxiety for the group therapist. Manifestations of countertransference can assume many forms not limited to feelings of inadequacy (McWilliams and Stein, 1987), boredom (Steichen, 1996), anger and hatred (Epstein, 1979; Gans, 1989; Hahn, 1995; Kirman, 1995), fear of abandonment or engulfment (HarPaz, 1994), and the helpless loss of control over the group (Ormont, 1991).

Winnicott (1949) was the first to coin the term "objective countertransference," referring to "the analyst's love and hate in reaction to the actual personality and behavior of the patient, based on objective observation" (p. 70). Moreover, Winnicott suggested that while objective hate is justified, "the analyst must be prepared to bear the strain without expecting the patient to know anything that he is doing, perhaps over a long period of time" (Winnicott, 1949, p. 72). He stated that communication of his reactions is withheld for later use at the appropriate time, and that this demand would be impossible unless the analyst remains aware of the feelings. Since Winnicott's seminal paper (1949), others have refined the distinction between objective and subjective countertransference (Spotnitz, 1969; 1976; Margolis, 1978). While both are induced by the patient's transference feelings, are manifested in myriad ways, and vary in intensity from mild to intense, subjective countertransference involves a reawakening of early identifications and unresolved conflicts, the feelings which usually linger long after the hour (Margolis, 1978). "With subjective countertransference, our reaction is highly individual, idiosyncratic" (Ormont, 1991, p. 434). It is this form of countertransference that can lead to obstacles (i.e., counterresistance) to effective treatment. For countertransference to have utility, it must be "purged of its subjective element" (Spotnitz, 1976).

DISAVOWING ANGER

Although there is much literature to suggest that not only is therapist anger an inevitable but useful component of psychodynamically oriented treatment, there also exist powerful obstacles to the beginning group therapist's acknowledgment of anger in the member and in himself. "The unseasoned group leader, in particular, may fear that his patients will leave if they get angry" (Ormont, 1984, p. 555), resulting in a sense of failure. Group therapists and new members enter into an implicit agreement that group therapy will provide an opportunity for symptom relief at a minimum, and ideally enduring character change. A primary expectation of the group member in this tacit agreement is that "the group, and you as group therapist, are going to help me alleviate my suffering." To the group therapist, wanting to do right by the group members is the motivational underpinning of a professional and ethical responsibility to provide competent treatment, but to the novice this produces a special pressure stemming from feelings of self-doubt inherent in learning to be a psychotherapist (Jacobs, David, & Meyer, 1995). This self-idealized expectation of the therapist intermingles with the member's need to find an all-knowing, expert healer, leaving the therapist "vulnerable to failing to live up to the jointly created idealized expectations" (Hahn, 1995, p. 340). Because so much of the beginning therapist's sense of self is bound up in the need to feel competent and able, client reactions that are perceived to threaten this self-ideal can create considerable discomfort. This is manifested in a sense of failure and subsequent feelings of anger stemming from the shame inherent in perceived failures (Hahn, 1995). These feelings were evoked in the trainee who was defined by Mary in the preceding vignette as a novice, and Mary's contempt was barely disguised in her excusing the young therapist's perceived incompetence due to inexperience. The trainee, whose *raison d'etre* was to help others, remained silent, afraid to draw additional fire from Mary, or Ed who was smoldering in his chair. Even the senior therapist felt tempted to dilute the moment with an intellectualized interpretation. But what was most needed was not to stifle the mounting anger and aggression, but remove the resistance to its verbal expression.

It should be noted that while trepidation might be one response to group aggression, so might counter-aggression. As the above vignette unfolded, the trainee eventually broke her silence by asking the group

"How might the group help Mary cope with her angry feelings" leading to a great deal of averted glances by others as if to communicate "Why are you bringing me into this?" The trainee, who later acknowledged in supervision with some difficulty that she was angry at the group for not being more active in confronting Mary (the source of this trainee's considerable discomfort), was aggressively acting out her anger toward the group by putting them on the spot. She also admitted feeling angry at Mary for her shaming remarks about her lack of skill as a group therapist, and only later realized that she indirectly criticized Mary for expressing her anger, thus effectively shutting her down. Mary fell into silence until a few moments later the senior therapist asked Ed how he (the therapist) and the trainee could have avoided such poor leadership during this session. This not only elicited a response from Mary, who was only too eager to respond, but also Ed who was once again cut-off by Mary. Ed felt that the leaders could have asked Mary to allow time for others to respond as well as to point out to her how she makes others not want to include her. He expressed his anger at the leaders (predominantly the senior therapist) for not intervening sooner, and he expressed anger at Mary for her "constant attacking of others without examining her own issues." The senior therapist turned to Sol and asked how they had failed the group, to which Sol replied "By not helping Mary and Ed find a way to connect to each other without their anger." Eventually Mary and Ed were able to communicate more effectively, and had they not graduated necessitating their leaving the group, might even have gotten around to expressing their attraction for one another as well, which was evident in subsequent groups over the following months.

SUPERVISION DILEMMAS

The above discussion and clinical vignette illustrate the extreme difficulty novice group therapists have in facilitating the communication of aggressive feelings. I do not wish to elucidate the many techniques that could have been used in the above vignette, but I do wish to highlight some dilemmas for supervision, especially as they occur in a co-therapy relationship between supervisor and supervisee. Modeling could be said to have been used in the above vignette as the supervisor modeled one method for not only facilitating the expression of anger, but also bringing more than one member into emotional contact with another and the leader, and directing anger away from a potential scapegoat (Mary) and onto the therapist. While on the one hand this served to illustrate technique, as well as demonstrate that the therapist can survive aggressive verbal communication in group, it did little to demonstrate that this trainee could also "do" and "survive" in the same manner. One way in which the supervisor in a co-therapy relationship can handle such a situation is to reveal her own feelings about a group exchange as the one described above. This does not mean to delve right into self-disclosure in the next supervisory session, but for the supervisor to judiciously model exploration and disclosure of her own countertransference communicates that this is an appropriate and acceptable activity in group psychotherapy supervision.

Countertransference exploration is central to any psychodynamically oriented supervision (Jacobs et al., 1995; Rock, 1997). Rock (1997) states that how countertransference is defined will dictate how it is dealt with in therapy and supervision. He suggests that supervisors use the totalistic definition of countertransference as encompassing all of the therapist's reactions to the patient, thus shifting the focus to the supervisee's subjective experience of the patient in the therapeutic interaction and away from the supervisee's problems. Fosshage (1997) goes further to emphasize a focus upon not just the experience of the patient, but also the experience of the session, including the interactions and emotional communication between the patient and therapist. In this manner, the impact of therapist (both the supervisor and supervisee) interventions can be monitored in addition to understanding of member dynamics. Facilitating self-reflection and revelation in a manner that engages curiosity about one's countertransference, protects the self-esteem of the supervisee, and communicates interest and aliveness in the supervisory relationship, reduces the activation of shame that can occur when critical or judgmental supervisory interventions are experienced as abrupt and threatening impingements to the supervisee's internal experience (Jacobs et al., 1995). Through modeling of self-disclosure and self-reflection, the supervisor can hope that through the supervisee's partial identification with her she can facilitate this kind of attitude in her supervisee. "The student has to recognize that he will develop countertransference reactions to every patient he works with," and that to detect and understand these reactions, although uncomfortable at times, is essential (Spotnitz, 1976).

Another dilemma arising in the above vignette is the shame that arose when the trainee's interventions failed, and the senior therapist's produced therapeutic movement. One contributing factor to the trainee's inability to tolerate failure had to do with the few attempts she initially made to intervene in the group, such that the few times she ventured an intervention contributed to a small ratio of successful to unsuccessful interventions. The senior clinician by contrast seemed more successful in his interventions, in part because of experience, but also in part because of his willingness to actively engage the members in emotional exchanges, positive and negative. With the reticent trainee I have sometimes pondered aloud how I might take up less space to allow her to develop more (i.e., attempt more interventions). With one supervisee this led to a fruitful discussion about how to follow-up on her interventions which would (a) communicate to her and the group members my valuing of her activity in the group; and (b) help her refine and hone her skills. In the above vignette, the group therapist might have said "I think Anne (the trainee) brings up a good point about how the group might help Mary. I guess I am wondering how Anne and I failed to bring this about." Asking the object oriented question as a follow-up to Anne's more critical intervention still supports her presence and activity in the group, but takes the burden off the egos of the group members and leads to removing resistance to the communication of anger in the group (Margolis, 1983), as well as models technique through refinement of her original intervention.

A final strategy that can help the trainee appreciate the challenges but rewards of attending to group member aggression, is through didactic readings and seminars that highlight the importance of unblocking the communication of aggression in groups; detecting and understanding our own aggressive impulses, especially in reaction to being targeted by group members for the expression of their anger; and lastly managing other countertransference reactions that might arise in reaction to group members' anger. Many of the readings reviewed here could go a long way in helping the trainee in group psychotherapy adopt an attitude of acceptance of the expression of aggression as a necessary means to maturational development. Moreover, accepting the inevitability of being the object of intense anger and even hatred from time to time, and having a theoretical island on which to stand and evaluate the maelstrom that often emerges when the group is storming, can provide tools to the developing group therapist for managing strong countertransference. In fact, supporting the clinical and theoretical literature is some empirical support for the reliance upon a theoretical framework lessening the extent to which therapists act out countertransference (Latts & Gelso, 1995; Robbins & Jolkovski, 1987). Having a theoretical port in the storm, combined with a supervisory relationship that is safe enough to allow exploration of countertransference, are key ingredients to helping the developing group therapist work with strong affect in groups.

CONCLUSIONS

Group therapists in training must come to terms with the fact that not only does anger and aggression flourish in group psychotherapy, but that the very nature of group psychotherapy facilitates its build-up (Ormont, 1984). Moreover, many patients seek treatment because they have established defenses to their own aggressive impulses, and these pent up feelings and impulses lead to significant blocks in maturational development (Spotnitz, 1976). When aggression emerges in group, especially when it becomes contagious within the membership, the leader is most often the appropriate target for its first significant expression. For the novice group therapist, this often runs counter to his idealized altruistic self-expectations (Hahn, 1995). The understandable urge is to restore a calm and respectful focus in our groups that exudes compassion and hope for each and every member. But what if this is inconsistent with the maturational needs of the client? Quite often this is the case, and what is needed maturationally is the unblocking of obstacle to the expression of aggression (Spotnitz, 1976). Although the focus of this paper was not to explore the many techniques useful for accomplishing this, the literature is replete with sources that not only expound on techniques for eliciting aggression in groups, but also how to judiciously communicate the therapist's "objective hatred" to clients consistent with their maturational needs (Epstein, 1979; Hahn, 1995; Spotnitz, 1976; Winnicott, 1949).

The developing group therapist needs to be able to detect her countertransference reactions to expressed aggression and use her own self-reflection and supervision to attempt to understand her feelings and their subjective elements. She must also appreciate how these feelings can offer valuable information through which to understand the group members. The extent to which group psychotherapy trainees are able to accomplish this task depends upon: (a) the ability of the supervisor to appreciate the potential for elicited shame when helping the supervisee reveal her personal reactions and feelings (Jacobs et al., 1995); (b) the degree of clinical and theoretical understanding the novice has about the role of aggression in groups; (c) the theoretical and clinical appreciation of the role of countertransference in group psychotherapy; and (d) the experience of witnessing how skillfully facilitated verbal expression of aggression can lead to maturational development in group members. A co-therapist relationship between a supervisor and a supervisee provides unique opportunities for the modeling of skills, the facilitation of self-reflection and self-revelation, and the partial identification to the supervisor in her role as a skilled group therapist

REFERENCES

Agazarian, Y. M. (1994). The phases of development and the system's-centered group. In M. Pines & V. Schermer (Eds.), Ring of fire: primitive object relations and affect in group psychotherapy. London: Routledge, Chapman & Hall.

Agazarian, Y. M. (1996). Systems-centered therapy for groups. New York: Guilford Press.

Arlow, J. A. (1985). Some technical problems of countertransference. *Psychoanalytic Quarterly, 54*, 164-174.

Bennis, W. G. & Shepard, H. A. (1956). A theory of group development. *Human Relations, 9*(4), 415-437.

Blanck, G. & Blanck, R. (1979). Ego psychology II: Psychoanalytic developmental psychology. New York: Columbia University Press.

Epstein, L. (1979). The therapeutic function of hate in the countertransference. In L. Epstein & A. Feiner (eds.), Countertransference (pp. 214-234). Northvale, NJ: Jason Aronson.

Fosshage, J. L. (1997). Toward a model of psychoanalytic supervision from a self psychological/intersubjective perspective. In M. H. Rock (Ed.), Psychodynamic supervision: Perspectives of the supervisor and the supervisee (pp. 105-132). Northvale, NJ: Jason Aronson.

Freud, S. (1910). Future prospects of psychoanalytic psychotherapy. In J. Strachey (Ed. and Trans.) (1959). The standard edition of the complete works of Sigmund Freud (Vol. 11, pp. 139-151). London: Hogarth.

Fromm-Reichmann, F. (1950). Principles of intensive psychotherapy. Chicago: University of Chicago Press.

Gabbard, G. O. (1989). Patients who hate. *Psychiatry, 52*, 96-106.

Gans, J. E. (1989). Hostility in group psychotherapy. *International Journal of Group Psychotherapy, 39*, 499-516

Gelso, C. J. & Carter, J. (1985). The relationship in counseling and psychotherapy. *The Counseling Psychologist, 13,* 155-244.

Grotjahn, M. (1953). Special aspects of countertransference in analytic group psychotherapy. *International Journal of Group Psychotherapy, 3,* 407-416.

Hahn, W. K. (1995). Therapist anger in group psychotherapy. *International Journal of group Psychotherapy, 45,* 339-347.

HarPaz, N. (1994). Failures in group psychotherapy: The therapist variable. *International Journal of Group Psychotherapy, 44,* 3-19.

Heiman, P. (1950). On countertransference. *International Journal of Psychoanalysis, 31,* 81 84.

Jacobs, D., David, P., & Meyer, D. J. (1995). The supervisory encounter: A guide for teachers of psychodynamic psychotherapy and psychoanalysis. New Haven: Yale University Press.

Kernberg, O. F. (1975). Borderline conditions and pathological narcissism. New York: Jason Aronson.

Kirman, J. H. (1995). Working with anger in groups: A modern analytic approach. *International Journal of Group Psychotherapy, 45,* 303-329.

Latts, M. G. & Gelso, C. J. (1995). Countertransference behavior and management with survivors of sexual assault. *Psychotherapy: Theory, Research, and Practice, 32,* 405-415.

Livingston, M. S. & Livingston, L. R. (1998). Conflict and aggression in group psychotherapy: A self psychological vantage point. *International Journal of Group Psychotherapy, 48,* 381-391.

Margolis, B.D. (1978). Narcissistic countertransference: Emotional availability and case management. *Modern Psychoanalysis, 3,* 133-151.

Margolis, B. D. (1983). The object oriented question: A contribution to treatment technique. *Modern Psychoanalysis, 8,* 35-46.

McWilliams, N. & Stein, J. (1987). Women's groups led by women: The management of devaluing transferences. *International Journal of Group Psychotherapy, 37,* 139-153.

Ormont, L. R. (1984). The leader's role in dealing with aggression in groups. *International Journal of Group Psychotherapy, 34,* 553-572.

Ormont, L. R. (1990). The craft of bridging. *International Journal of Group Psychotherapy, 40,* 3-17.

Ormont, L. R. (1991). Use of the group in resolving the subjective countertransference. *International Journal of Group Psychotherapy, 41,* 433-447.

Ormont, L. R. (1997). Bridging in group analysis. *Modern Psychoanalysis, 22,* 59-77.

Peabody, S. A. & Gelso, C. J. (1982). Countertransference and empathy: The complex relationship between two divergent concepts in counseling. *Journal of Counseling Psychology, 29,* 240-245.

Reich, A. (1951). On countertransference. *International Journal of Psychoanalysis, 32,* 25-31.

Reich, A. (1960). Further remarks on countertransference. *International Journal of Psychoanalysis, 41,* 389-395.

Robbins, S. B. & Jolkovski, M. P. (1987). Managing countertransference feelings: An interactional model using awareness of feelings and theoretical framework. *Journal of Counseling Psychology, 34,* 276-282.

Rock, M. H. (1997). Effective supervision. In M. H. Rock (Ed.), Psychodynamic supervision: Perspectives of the supervisor and the supervisee (pp. 105-132). Northvale, NJ: Jason Aronson.

Rosenthal, L. (1987). Resolving resistance in group psychotherapy. Northvale, NJ: Jason Aronson.

Slavson, S. R. (1957). Are there "group dynamics" in therapy groups? *International Journal of Group Psychotherapy, 7,* 131-154.

Spotnitz, H. (1969). *Modern psychoanalysis of the schizophrenic patient.* New York: Grune & Stratton.

Spotnitz, H. (1976). *Psychotherapy of preoedipal conditions: Schizophrenia and severe character disorders.* New York: Jason Aronson.

Steichen, J. (1996). The modern group psychoanalytic use of countertransference as a tool for enhancing empathy and growth. *Modern Group, 1,* 85-96.

Winnicott, D. W. (1949). Hate in the countertransference. *The International Journal of Psycho-analysis, 30,* 69-74.

Yalom, I. (1975). The theory and practice of group psychotherapy (2nd ed.). New York: Basic Books.

An Introduction to the Internet
for Independent Group Therapists

Ralph Cafolla

SUMMARY. In the past several years, the growth of the Internet and World Wide Web has caused professionals in all occupations, including independent group therapists, to seek ways to use this new technology in the workplace. The purpose of this paper is to provide independent group therapists with a brief overview of the Internet and the World Wide Web and how it can be used to enhance their professional practices. The first part uses a question and answer format to present a brief overview of the Internet, including a discussion of the hardware and software needed to get on-line. The second part focuses on the uses of the Internet for communication and research for practicing health professionals. *[Article copies available for a fee from The Haworth Document Delivery Service: 1-800-342-9678. E-mail address: getinfo@haworthpressinc.com <Website: http://www.haworthpressinc.com>]*

KEYWORDS. Group psychotherapy, Internet, independent/private practice/practitioners

INTRODUCTION

The Internet has evolved in the past three years from a toy for the technological elite to an important form of communication and infor-

---

Dr. Cafolla served on the faculties of Florida International University, the City University of New York and Barry University. He is currently Associate Professor in the Department of Educational Technology and Research at Florida Atlantic University. Dr. Cafolla is an international lecturer who has written two books and numerous papers on the uses of the World Wide Web and related technologies.

[Haworth co-indexing entry note]: "An Introduction to the Internet for Independent Group Therapists." Cafolla, Ralph. Co-published simultaneously in *Journal of Psychotherapy in Independent Practice* (The Haworth Press, Inc.) Vol. 1, No. 2, 2000, pp. 77-86; and: *Group Therapy in Independent Practice* (ed: Scott Simon Fehr) The Haworth Press, Inc., 2000, pp. 77-86. Single or multiple copies of this article are available for a fee from The Haworth Document Delivery Service [1-800-342-9678, 9:00 a.m. - 5:00 p.m. (EST). E-mail address: getinfo@haworthpressinc.com].

mation for everyone. More and more professionals are finding it an important source for information in their fields. The purpose of this paper is to provide independent group therapists with a brief overview of the Internet and the World Wide Web and how it can be used to enhance their professional practices. The paper is divided into two parts. The first part uses a question and answer format to present a brief overview of the Internet, including a discussion of the hardware and software needed to get on-line. The second part focuses on the uses of the Internet for communication and research for practicing health professionals.

INTERNET FREQUENTLY ASKED QUESTIONS

On the Internet, many sites use a question and answer format to answer questions that users ask often. In telecommunications jargon, these are called Frequently Asked Questions or FAQs. As the name implies, this section will use this format to present some of the more commonly asked questions about the Internet and provide brief answers.

WHAT IS THE INTERNET?

The Internet is commonly referred to as the information superhighway, and in many ways the analogy is valid. The Internet was designed by the United States government during the Cold War as a means of assuring that the many computers in military installations could communicate with each other in time of war. Interestingly, the Interstate Highway system was constructed in the prior decade for much the same reason. While a detailed explanation of how the Internet works is beyond the scope of this paper, it is sufficient to say that the Internet is a group of technologies designed to allow computers to talk to each other. This technology consists of hardware (computers, telephone lines, and so forth) and sets of rules or protocols (called *Internet Protocols* or *IPs*).

One of the first uses of the Internet was electronic mail, or e-mail. E-mail allows you to send personal messages to each other even though they may have accounts on different computers. E-mail is also the basis for electronic discussion forums called listservs. While e-mail is directed to a specific person, a letter to a listserv is sent to all listserv users. In general, people with common interests (like group therapy) would join a listserv to communicate with others with the same interest. The use of listservs by independent group counselors is discussed later. Other early Internet services included a set of rules (called *File Transfer Protocols* or *FTP*) to allow the transfer of files over the Internet and *telnet,* which allowed you to sign on to any computer on the Internet from any other computer. In the early days, only real computer geeks could learn how to use all of the services provided by the Internet. Then came the World Wide Web.

WHAT IS THE WORLD WIDE WEB?

The World Wide Web (or simply, the Web) was designed by scientists to make the Internet easier to use by uniting all of the Internet services into a common interface. The key to this simplicity was the use of a hypertext interface. Hypertext allows certain words in a document to act as links to other parts of the document or, in fact, any location on the Internet. The hypertext links have a distinctive appearance on the document and the user selects the text by pointing and clicking with the mouse.

One of the most appealing facets of the Web is the ease with which one can create a document, called a Web page. There are computer programs, many available for free, that are almost as easy to use as a word processor. This fact has enabled many people in non-computer related professions, including therapists, to establish a presence on the Web. Whether you want to just use the Web to get information or are interested in your own Web page, there are certain computer hardware and software items you will need.

WHAT DO I NEED TO CONNECT?

The two basic components of going on-line are the computer and the telephone. One also needs a device that converts, or modulates, the digital output of the computer into an analog format that can be sent over regular telephone lines. This device, which must also demodulate (convert back from the analog phone signal to digital input on the receiving computer) is called a *Modulator/Demodulator* or *modem.* All modern computers come equipped with a high-speed (56K) modem as part of the basic package. If you are uncomfortable with a computer, you can also use your regular television with WebTV. This service provides Internet access without the use of a computer. All you need is your television and a keyboard that WebTV provides. Obviously, this solution, while easier to use, is not as flexible as a real computer. In addition, with the prices of high powered computers so low, it seems advisable to use the computer to access the Internet.

Once you have the hardware, you will need to find a company to sell you Internet services, much as your cable company sells you a television signal. These companies are known as *Internet Service Providers,* or *ISP*s. There are hundreds of such companies in the country, so finding one in your area should be relatively easy. Many large national companies like AT&T, MCI, and America Online also provide Internet connections. These companies will also provide you with whatever software you need to connect. This will include the basic software, called a browser, needed to access the Web. Internet Explorer and Netscape, both available at no cost, are two of the most popular browsers. Now that you know what the Internet is and how to get on-line, you probably want to know what a group therapist might do with it.

THE INTERNET AND INDEPENDENT GROUP THERAPISTS

In the 1960s, Marshall McLuhan (1964) suggested that media was an extension of the body: the telephone an extension of the ear and mouth, the television of the eyes, and so forth. He used the term *Global Village* to describe a world linked by satellites and other technologies that would allow everyone in the world to know what everyone else was doing. His theory was right, but the technology was wrong–the Web, not network television, is the Global Village. The mass media of yesterday has given way to a more narrow, person-to-person technology. The Web is an extension of your ability to communicate; an important function of the therapist. The next section discusses how therapists can use the Web to improve communications with both colleagues and patients.

ELECTRONIC MAIL (E-MAIL)

Electronic mail, or e-mail, occupies a unique place in the world of communications. Faster than the regular post office (derisively called "snail mail" by Internet mavens) yet not as instantaneous as a telephone call, e-mail, like most other Internet services, is becoming ever more popular and easy to use. You would probably be surprised to find out how many of your patients and colleagues have and use e-mail on a regular basis. Like other forms of communication you might provide patients, there are some issues to be considered.

One issue that is fairly obvious is the question of just how available you want to be. Some therapists give patients their home telephone numbers and some do not. You might consider that one advantage of e-mail is that you check it at your convenience. Perhaps by providing patients with this method of communication, they would be less likely to call. It is also important to consider what types of e-mail you would encourage. You might want to limit it to business issues, like changing an appointment. You certainly would not want to open yourself to giving "round the clock" therapy. You might not want to let your patients contact you via e-mail at all. In that case, it can still be a useful way to communicate with colleagues. E-mail is informal and provides a convenient way of sharing ideas and concerns.

Most e-mail programs also allow you to set up distribution lists. This permits you to send mail to a group of people at one time. For example, you could have a list called "Monday Men's Group," and broadcast a message to all the members at once. Since it is unlikely that all of your patients have and use e-mail, this form of communication must be viewed as an addition to rather than a replacement for more traditional forms of communications.

USING LISTSERVS

E-mail also serves as the basis for electronic forums called listservs. These provide a forum for people with similar interests to share ideas. As independent therapists, it may be difficult to find fellow professionals with whom to discuss issues. Because listservs have no geographical boundaries, you can communicate with therapists all over the world. Because it is based on e-mail, you can participate as much as you wish. For example, the American Psychological Association (APA) sponsors a group psychotherapy forum. Members of this forum are able to post messages and discuss matters relevant to issues in group psychotherapy with their colleagues. Joining the group psychotherapy listserv is easy: Just send an e-mail message to listserv@

lisp.apa.org. The message should consist of the following lines. SUB-SCRIBE GROUP-PSYCHOTHERAPY YourFirstName YourLastName END (Note: you should leave the Subject: (or To:) field blank if your e-mail program will let you.) Within a short time, you will be con-firmed as a member of the listserv and will be able to participate in the conversation. If the e-mail address should change by the time of the publishing of this journal, it is quite easy to find the new e-mail address by simply going into your search engine and typing Group Therapy. Your search engine will give you the new URL. All you have to do is click on it.

In addition to using the Web to enhance communications, it is also a major source of information in your professional practice. The balance of this paper will present some sources of information for group thera-pists and describe how you can find additional resources.

RESEARCH

In the old days (about three years ago) finding current information in your field meant subscribing to expensive journals or making fre-quent trips to the library. Now, thanks to the World Wide Web, you can find a vast amount of up-to-date information with a click of the mouse. You will, of course, need some starting points. Web sites are addressed using what is called a *Uniform Resource Locator* or *URL*. These URLs usually look like this:

http://www.something.something

For example, the APA Web site is: http://www.apa.org and is read:

www dot apa dot org

You access a Web site by getting on the Internet, starting your Web browser, and typing the URL in the *address* box. Below is a brief description of some useful Web sites for practicing psychologists along with their URLs.

SOME USEFUL SITES

As noted above, American Psychological Association (APA) main-tains a large Web site (*http://www.apa.org*). It is mostly for members, but it has a large, free public area. The site has an on-line edition of the *APA Monitor,* which contains informative stories on what is happening in psychology. Members also have access to *PsycINFO,* an electronic database of abstracts on over 1,350 scholarly journals. The Help Center provides up-to-date information on dealing with life problems. The site also povides a wealth of public information related to psychology.

The Mental Health Net *(http://www.cmhc.com/),* which claims to be the definitive guide to mental health, psychology, and psychiatry resources online, currently indexes over 8,000 referred resources. You can find updated information for just about any psychological disorder you can think of. You will also find links to various mental health organizations.

Mentalhealth.com's *(http://www.mentalhealth.com/)* goal is to improve understanding, diagnosis, and treatment of mental illness throughout the world. You can look up any of the fifty-two (52) most common mental disorders and find a description, diagnosis, treatment and research findings for each. There is also information about the most common psychiatric drugs including indications, contraindications, warnings, precautions, adverse effects, overdose, dosage, and research findings. There is also an extensive list of mental health links

The Mental Health Source *(http://www.mhsource.com/)* provides the latest news, special offers, upcoming meetings and classified practice opportunities listed by state, residency, fellowships, products, office space and more. You can also find pointers to the MHI Professional Directory that lists mental health professionals geographically. You can also obtain your own directory listing.

Psych Central *(http://psychcentral.com/),* maintained by Dr. John Grohol, attempts to be a one-stop index for psychology, support, mental health issues, resources, and people on the Internet. This resource is updated regularly and has been featured in *The Wall Street Journal, Newsweek, U.S. News & World Report,* the *Washington Post, USA Today, The Village Voice, Business Week* and dozens of other publications. This site contains pointers to newsgroups

Two other sites, Psyc Link *(http://www.psychlink.com/)* and Networked Resources in Psychology and Mental Health *(http://plaza. interport.net/nypsan/network.html)* are useful because of their extensive pointers to Mental Health web resources. These resources include research organizations and facilities, colleges and universities, journals and newsletters, and newsgroups. Also available are links to publishers and clearinghouses, listservs and subscription services and other useful mental health resources.

While these Web sites provide a good starting point and also have many links to other psychology related sites, once you become familiar with the Web, you will want to find your own resources. The next section discusses how you can search the Internet on your own.

SEARCHING THE INTERNET

The ease of creating Web sites has led to a proliferation of information available on the Web. This is both good news and bad. The odds are that the information you want is somewhere on the Web, but finding it makes the proverbial search for a "needle in a haystack" seem trivial. Luckily, the Web has powerful tools called *search engines* to help you. These engines, found at various locations on the Web, use artificial intelligence techniques to search through the mountains of sites on the Web. There are basically two types of search engines, indexes and free searches.

Yahoo *(http://www.yahoo.com)* is an example of a hypertext based index to the Web. If you are searching for a broad category, this method works quite well. For example, navigating from the Yahoo Home to the Health sections will lead you to a Health Psychology page. You can then follow the hyperlinks to additional resources.

Alta Vista *(http://www.altavista.com)* excels at free searches of the Web. If you are looking for something very specific, this type of search engine may be best. You simply type in the word or words that you want to search for and Alta Vista takes over. For instance, a search on the phrase "group therapy" yielded 233,690 hits. Admittedly, many of these will not be what you are looking for, but there is sure to be some interesting information.

WEAVING YOUR OWN WEB PAGE

As noted above, it is easy to create your own Web pages. Web editing programs are easy to use and can be mastered in a few hours. While you do have to understand the basic terminology of the Web, there is no computer programming needed. You simply type in the same way you would a word processor. Typical word processing features such as cut-and-paste and text formatting commands are available and you are working in a What You See Is What You Get (WYSI-WYG–pronounced "Wizzy-Wig") environment. Inserting pictures and hyperlinks is accomplished with a click of a mouse. Two of the best Web editors are absolutely free–in fact they are part of both the Netscape Communicator and Internet Explorer browser programs. You can download the software from either *http://www.netscape.com* or *http://www.microsoft.com*. Front Page Express is the program that is now part of Explorer, while Netscape Composer comes bundled with Communicator.

Once you have created your Web pages, you are ready to put them on the Web. Many times, your Internet Service Provider (ISP) give you free Web space. If they don't, no problem. There are several commercial companies that provide free space on their Web site. The only downside is that the pages are accompanied by some advertising (someone has to pay!). Two of the more popular of these free sites are Geocities *(http://www.geocities.com)* and Xoom *(http://www.xoom.com)*. You can visit their site to learn more about the services they offer.

CONCLUSION

The Internet and the World Wide Web provide access to communications and information for professionals in many disciplines. With just a modest investment in time and money, the independent group therapist can tap the power of the Internet to enhance his or her practice.

REFERENCES

Alta Vista Corporation Home Page, [On-line]. Available: http://www.altavista.com
American Psychological Association, [On-line]. Available: http://www.apa.org/
Link, (1998), Home Page, [On-line]. Available: http://www.psychlink.com/
McLuhan, M., (1964). *Understanding media: the extensions of man,* McGraw-Hill: New York.
Mentalhealth.com's. [On-line]. Available: http://www.mentalhealth.com/
Mental Health Net, [On-line]. Available: http://www.cmhc.com/
Mental Health Source, [On-line]. Available: http://www.mhsource.com/
Netscape Corporation, (1998), Home Page, [On-line]. Available: http://www.netscape.com

Networked Resources in Psychology and Mental Health, (1998), Home Page, [On-line]. Available: http://plaza.interport.net/nypsan/network.html

Psych Central, (1998), Home Page, [On-line]. Available: http://psychcentral.com/Psyc

Xoom, (1998), Home Page, [On-line]. Available: http://www.xoom.com

Yahoo Search Engine, (1998), Home Page, [On-line]. Available: http://www.yahoo.com

Index

Abandonment (feelings of), 66
Activity analysis of group process, 21-32
Adderall, 55
ADHD. *See* Attention Deficit Disorder with Hyperactivity (ADHD)
Adolescents
  Attention Deficit Disorder with Hyperactivity (ADHD) in. *See* Attention Deficit Disorder with Hyperactivity (ADHD)
  benefits of group psychotherapy, 53
  Conduct Disorder, 54
  identity development, 53-62
  Oppositional Defiant Disorder, 54
  shame (feelings of), 53-54,57-59,61
Affective disorders, 3
Agazarian, Y.M., 64-65
Aggression (feelings of), 15,64,66, 71-72
AGPA. *See* American Group Psychotherapy Association (AGPA)
Akron Child Guidance Center, 33
Allusion, literary, 4-7
Alonso, A., 15
Alta Vista (Internet search engine), 84
Ambivalence (feelings of), 64
America Online (Internet Service Provider), 80
American Group Psychotherapy Association (AGPA), 3,13, 43,45-46
American Occupational Therapy Association (AOTA), 22-26
American Psychological Association (APA), 81-83
Analytic therapy groups, 13-19
Anger (feelings of), 8,19,34,38,63-75

Anxiety (feelings of), 8,14,18,64,67
AOTA. *See* American Occupational Therapy Association (AOTA)
APA. *See* American Psychological Association (APA)
APA Monitor, 83
Arlow, J.A., 66
AT&T (Internet Service Provider), 80
Attention Deficit Disorder with Hyperactivity (ADHD)
  benefits of group psychotherapy with adolescents, 53-57,60
  defined, 53-54
  group psychotherapy vs. individual therapy, 53-55
  group therapy methods, 59-60
  identity issues in adolescents with, 54-62
  medications, use of, 55

Barkley, R.A., 54,57
Barnes, M.A., 2,21
Barry University, 77 ˙
Beck, A.P., 15
Behavioral methods of group psychotherapy, 21-22
Beit-Berl College, 43
Benefits of group psychotherapy, 1-2
Bennis, W.G., 64-65
Bereavement groups, 33-41
Bion, W., 45
Blanck, G., 67
Blanck, R., 67
Borderline personality disorders, 6
Boredom (feelings of), 67
Boston Institute of Psychotherapy, 3
Boston School of Occupational Therapy, Tufts University, 21
Brothers Karamazov, The, 5

defined, 64
multiple transference relationships,
67
transference-countertransference
interactions, 63-75
Tufts University, Boston School of
Occupational Therapy, 21

UMASS Adolescent Inpatient
Program, Westboro,
Massachusetts, 21
Uniform terminology for occupational
therapy, 24f-25f
Universality, 7
University of Maryland, Counseling
Psychology Program, 63

Van Wagoner, S., 2,63
Vinogradov, S., 38-40

Washington Square Institute, 13
Web sites
American Psychological
Association, 82-83
creating, 84-85
Mental Health Net, 83
Mental Health Source, 83
Mental Health, 83-84
MentalHealth.com, 83
Networked Resources in
Psychology and Mental
Health, 83-84
Psych Central, 83
Psych Link, 83-84
PsycINFO, 83
Webster, D., 22
WebTV, 79-80
Weinberg, H., 432
Wexler, D., 59
Willy Loman (literary character), 5
Wilson, E., 34
Winnicott, D.W., 67,72
World Wide Web (WWW), 77-86. *See
also* Internet. *See also* Web
sites
WWW. *See* World Wide Web (WWW)

Yahoo (Internet search engine), 84
Yalom, I.D., 7,15,27,34,38-40,
44-45,59-60,64-65

T - #0154 - 270225 - C0 - 212/152/6 - PB - 9780789010346 - Gloss Lamination